P9-DZN-603

Springer Series on **ADULTHOOD and AGING**

Volume 1 Adult Day Care: Community Work with the Elderly
Philip G. Weiler and Eloise Rathbone-McCuan, with contributors

Volume 2 Counseling Elders and Their Families: Practical Techniques for Applied Gerontology
John J. Herr and John H. Weakland

Volume 3 Becoming Old: An Introduction to Social Gerontology
John C. Morgan

Volume 4 The Projective Assessment of Aging Method (PAAM)
Bernard D. Starr, Marcella Bakur Weiner, and Marilyn Rabetz

Volume 5 Ethnicity and Aging
Donald E. Gelfand and Alfred J. Kutzik, with 25 contributors

Volume 6 Gerontology Instruction in Higher Education
David A. Peterson and Christopher R. Bolton

Volume 7 Nontraditional Therapy and Counseling with the Aging
S. Stansfeld Sargent, with 18 contributors

Volume 8 The Aging Network: Programs and Services, 2nd ed.
Donald E. Gelfand

Volume 9 Old Age on the New Scene
Robert Kastenbaum, with 29 contributors

Volume 10 Controversial Issues in Gerontology
Harold J. Wershow, with 36 contributors

Volume 11 Open Care for the Aging: Comparative International Approaches
Virginia C. Little

Volume 12 The Older Person as a Mental Health Worker
Rosemary McCaslin, with 11 contributors

Volume 13 The Elderly in Rural Society: Every Fourth Elder
Raymond T. Coward and Gary R. Lee, with 16 contributors

Volume 14 Social Support Networks and the Care of the Elderly: Theory, Research, and Practice
William J. Sauer and Raymond T. Coward, with 17 contributors

Volume 15: Managing Home Care for the Elderly: Lessons from Community-based Agencies
Anabel O. Pelham and William F. Clark, with 10 contributors

Anabel O. Pelham, Ph.D., is currently Director of Gerontology Programs in Extended Education at San Francisco State University. She received her degree from the University of California, San Francisco. Her professional experiences include academic program development and teaching in gerontology, older adult education program development, and university administration. Dr. Pelham has written on medical sociology, qualitative methods in field research, aging policy, and gerontology, and is co-author of *Old and Poor: A Study of Low Income Elderly and the Continuum of Care*. She is a member of the Social Policy and Long-Term Care sections of the American Society on Aging. Her current research interests include aging social and health policy, the social construction of aging, and applied gerontology. Dr. Pelham resides in San Francisco and is a collector of Northern California Chardonnay wines.

William F. Clark, M.P.P., served in the Peace Corps in Peru for eight years before entering graduate school. After receiving his degree in public policy from the University of California, Berkeley, in 1976, he continued public service with the State of California. Currently, he is Research Director for the Multipurpose Senior Services Program of the California Department of Aging. Mr. Clark has written on widowhood among low income elderly and their informal support systems, and is co-author of *Old and Poor: A Study of Low Income Elderly and the Continuum of Care*. He is an instructor at San Francisco State University, where he teaches aging policy courses. Mr. Clark's primary research is in the delivery of services to low income elders. He also retains his interest in pre-Columbian art and cultures.

MANAGING HOME CARE FOR THE ELDERLY

Lessons from Community-based Agencies

Anabel O. Pelham, Ph.D.
William F. Clark, M.P.P.
Editors

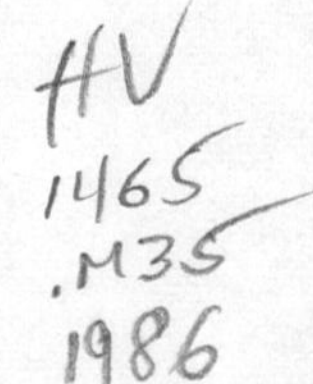

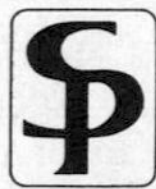

SPRINGER PUBLISHING COMPANY
New York

To our parents

Springer Publishing Company, Inc.
536 Broadway
New York, New York 10012

86 87 88 89 90 / 10 9 8 7 6 5 4 3 2 1

Library of Congress Cataloging-in-Publication Data

Main entry under title:
Managing home care for the elderly.
(Springer series on adulthood and aging; v. 15)
Bibliography: p. Includes index.
1. Aged—Home Care—United States—Addresses, essays, lectures.
2. Long-term care facilities—United States—Addresses, essays, lectures.
3. Aged—Services for—United States—Addresses, essays, lectures. 4. Aged—Government policy—United States—Addresses, essays, lectures. I. Pelham, Anabel O. II. Clark, William F. III. Series.
HV1465.M35 1985 362.6'3 85-12671
ISBN 0-8261-4700-3

Printed in the United States of America

Contents

Contributors

Richard Browdie, M.B.A., began his career as a caseworker in 1970, and initiated the development of services for the elderly in rural Erie County, Pennsylvania. After several years of planning and development roles, he became the first Director of the Erie County Area Agency on Aging. In 1979 he joined the newly formed Pennsylvania Department of Aging. Subsequently he assumed his current position as Deputy Executive Director of the Philadelphia Corporation for Aging.

Betty Havens, M.A., is Provincial Gerontologist for the Manitoba Department of Health. Her research specialty is matching assessed needs with effective community resources, especially through community-based home care policies. She is also a past president of the Canadian Association on Gerontology.

Becky Peters, R.N., is currently administering a private community-based long-term care agency in Santa Cruz, California called LIFESPAN: CARE MANAGEMENT FOR ELDERS. Ms. Peters received her degree from the Medical University of South Carolina. She has six years of experience in geriatric nursing and teaches in the Cabrillo College Gerontology Program in Santa Cruz.

Joan L. Quinn, R.N., M.S.N., is President of Connecticut Community Care, Inc. and former Executive Director of Triage, Inc. She is a nationally-recognized consultant on case management and long-term care. She is the author of numerous books and articles, has testified frequently in Washington, D.C., and consults regularly with policymakers throughout the United States. Ms. Quinn was recently presented with the American Nurses Association's Gerontological Nurse of the Year Award.

David W. Rieck, M.B.A., is Vice President of Connecticut Community Care, Inc. and former Assistant Director of Triage, Inc. Mr. Rieck has been instrumental in the development of statistical, financial, and administrative report systems which support the provision of long-term care to large populations of elderly persons. He has consulted frequently with developing organizations throughout the country.

Kirby G. Shoaf, M.B.A., is currently Executive Director of the Community Care Organization of Milwaukee County, Inc. He has also served as a mental health program director in Wisconsin as well as a nursing home and acute care hospital administrator in California.

Dennis Stone, M.D., is Director of Community Geriatric Medicine, Contra Costa County Health Services in California. He is also the Medical Director of Francis Nursing Home. Previously, for ten years he was the Medical Director for the North of Market Senior Service Center in San Francisco's Tenderloin district.

Adrian Turwoski, M.S.W., is presently a Social Services Advisor for the Oakland, California Multipurpose Senior Services Program. He also has developed and administered programs for the elderly in Pennsylvania, as well as taught case management practice and acted as a consultant.

Melvin J. Weinstein, M.S.W., is Director of Association for Services for the Aged, a 600-client Medicaid homecare program in Brooklyn, New York. Previously, he was Assistant Director of New York City's Department for the Aging's Home Care Project. A graduate of the State University of New York at Buffalo, Mr. Weinstein has served as technical consultant to various agencies including the Health Care Financing Administration and the YMCA of Greater New York.

Chana Zlotnick, M.Ed., M.S.W., is the Assistant Administrator of River Manor, a 380-bed health-related facility in Brooklyn, New York. She was formerly at the Albert Einstein College of Medicine as Site Coordinator of New York City's Department for the Aging's Home Care Project. Her experiences span community and institution-based practice, including development and management of adult day care. She has also taught courses in gerontology.

Preface

Community-based long-term care of the elderly is an ideal that is becoming a reality. Funded by the Health Care Financing Administration (HCFA) of the United States Department of Health and Human Services, research and demonstration projects in home care for the frail elderly have recently emerged across the United States. Similar social experiments are well under way in Canada.

Managing Home Care for the Elderly is a collection of essays that concern these projects and the human groups who attempt to care for their frail and elderly members at home. We see their efforts as societal actions to create "kinstitutions"—hybrid symbiotic kinship and institutional relationships. Community-based long-term care agencies are kinstitutions in every sense of the word. Their experience of struggling to become both family and formal organizations to frail elders promises to change the terrain of long-term care in the foreseeable future.

Acknowledgments

As with any scientific undertaking, this book was made possible through the efforts of many others. We would like to acknowledge the work of our contributors who labored to write about their adventures in practice and in organizing—while they were living it. Our thanks also go to Dr. Leonard Schatzman of the University of California at San Francisco for permission to employ his concept of kinstitution. Kinstitutions are indeed real. Our gratitude remains for all the research assistants in the California Senior Survey for opening their minds and hearts, and for honestly telling us how and what it was like to interview the poor elderly. We appreciate the patience and support of family, friends, and colleagues as we immersed ourselves in the time-consuming work of editing. Finally, our praise to Diann S. Haines who navigated the manuscript through typing, word processing, and final manuscript. Her extraordinary dedication and astute insights were of immeasurable value.

Introduction

Anabel O. Pelham and William F. Clark

THE EVOLUTION OF COMMUNITY-BASED LONG-TERM CARE

Community-based long-term care is a relatively recent phenomenon in the United States. As an organized and coherent approach to serving the elderly it is a little over a decade old. The new dimension of this approach is the *community-based* aspect which attempts to maintain frail elders at home. This differentiates it from the traditional approach which utilizes nursing homes to provide long-term care for the elderly. The developmental impetus for community-based long-term care was the explosive growth of nursing homes after the establishment of Medicare and Medicaid in 1965. Before 1965 the least fortunate elderly were cared for in public "poor houses" or in "Mom and Pop" operated "old folks" homes. This type of institutional bias is consistent with American social welfare policy and its philosophical origins in the English Poor Laws. These laws had an emphasis on "indoor" relief (e.g., poorhouse) in contrast to providing assistance in one's home.

With infusions of Medicare and Medicaid monies, nursing homes became a "growth industry." For example, in 1965 a total of $0.7 billion of public monies were expended on nursing home care in the United States, one-third of the total nursing home bill of $1.2 billion. In 1983, the total nursing home bill was $30.3 billion and the public share, now 55 percent, was $16.4 billion. The total bill for 1990 is projected to be $67.1 billion.

Most public financing of this growth comes from Medicaid, Title XIX of the Social Security Act, the principal public payer of health care for the poor of all ages. Medicaid is jointly funded by the states and the federal government can represent a sizeable component of a state's budget. For example, the Medicaid program in California, called Medi-Cal, represents about one-third of the total state budget. So, when a group of respected and humane professionals began advocating less expensive approaches to care for the elderly—approaches that would dampen the growth of nursing home expenditures—federal and state health care officials listened with avid interest.

Concurrent with these fiscal developments another phenomenon occurred: the well-publicized nursing home scandals of the 1970s. Unqualified providers, as well as real criminals, entered the nursing home field and soon scandalous "horror stories" appeared in the daily news. The tremendous infusion of monies happened before the federal or state governments could establish appropriate regulatory and licensure guidelines about who should be placed in nursing homes or what kind of care they should receive. Soon after horror stories appeared in the media, elected officials at all levels of government began a series of inquiries. Investigative hearings held in the early seventies brought out more stories of abuse and criminal behavior and led to legislative reforms.

In addition to reforms aimed at nursing homes per se (e.g., detailed licensing regulations and specific protocols for on-site inspections), various state legislatures authorized the search for alternatives to nursing home care. This search revealed that, at the local level, small nonprofit organizations had developed specific proposals for alternatives and, in a few cases, were implementing these on shoestring budgets. A few small pilot efforts had even been carried out a decade earlier (Katz et al., 1972).

In general, these alternatives took the form of a multidisciplinary team approach to caring for the elderly and providing the additional services necessary to keep the elder at home. The team was usually a nurse and a social worker who coordinated other providers. Given shared responsibility, the elder's physician played less of the traditionally dominant role. Supportive services were usually personal care (e.g., bathing and dressing) and chore services (e.g., housekeeping and meal preparation).

FUNDING AND THE ROLES OF THE HEALTH CARE FINANCING ADMINISTRATION

A major task during those early days was to secure funding for both additional services and new staffing configurations. After searching for various sources these new organizations concentrated on the Health Care Financing Administration (HCFA) and, to a lesser extent, on the Administration on Aging of the U.S. Department of Health and Human Services. HCFA is responsible for administering Medicaid and Medicare and for authorizing research and demonstration projects. Various projects, some of which are included in this volume, secured "waivers" which allowed them to use Medicaid or Medicare funds in nontraditional ways. In these cases, HCFA "waived" regulations which governed the usual and customary use of these funds.

What the various local and state entities proposed to HCFA was based on the premise that these alternative approaches would save money. Money would be saved since elderly clients served by these projects would avoid costly nursing home placements. Elders could receive less expensive but more appropriate care at home. Supporting the credibility of this money saving premise, proponents of these alternatives cited many studies which reported that large percentages of nursing home patients were inappropriately placed at this costly level of care. The argument was that these inappropriately placed persons could be served at home for a longer period at less cost with a better quality of life if only a few additional services were authorized.

During the 1970s HCFA funded 13 home care research and demonstration projects, all initiated at either the state or local level. The first one which was funded was Triage, Inc., in Connecticut in 1974. All together, nine states had projects, with the most (four) and the largest (the Multipurpose Senior Services Project) in California. Almost all of the projects have either been terminated or have been transformed into ongoing programs.

Even though preliminary evaluative results did not show overwhelming dollar savings—due to high administrative costs and to serving elders who were not at imminent risk of nursing home placements—the projects were otherwise politically successful. Elected officials of both parties renewed funding for these projects and authorized additional ones. The popularity of this community-based approach was such that in 1981 Congress included in the Omnibus Reconciliation Act a section which authorized states to initiate programs similar to the Medicaid-funded research and demonstration projects described in this volume. This piece of legislation is referred to as the Home and Community-Based Waivers or "2176 Waivers" (which designates the section number of the Omnibus Reconciliation Act where the waiver authorization appears).

It is interesting to note that this legislation was passed before any body of scientific literature had been created from the experiences of the research and demonstration projects. Although all projects had evaluation components attached to them, final results were often not available and Congress did not wait.

Another interesting aspect of this historical evolution has been the role played by HCFA. As the federal administrator of Medicare and Medicaid its Division of Long Term Care Experimentation was responsible for approving and overseeing the demonstration projects. More often than not, negotiations to obtain approval could literally take years as well as application of considerable political pressure. No doubt, from the federal perspective, the long drawn out approval process was productively used to winnow out ill-conceived projects or to improve the initial proposed design and planning process. From the point of view of the applicant, the lengthy process was detrimental to implementation since the applicant usually had to hold together a fragile coalition of groups and interests who were involved in the proposal. The longer the process the higher the chance that the coalition had of falling apart. Toward the late seventies officials of HCFA were even more reluctant to approve projects until its own initiated effort, referred to as "Channeling," could be implemented.

This effort by HCFA was an attempt to establish some federal leadership in the field of community-based long-term care in response to the innovations and initiatives coming from the state and local levels. In 1981, Congress passed the Home and Community-Based Waiver authority before any "Channeling" clients had been recruited. By July 1983, 33 states had had programs approved. However, demand for the Home and Community-Based Waivers is so great that the final results of the "Channeling" effort may be available only after all states have established programs.

HCFA's inability to directly contribute knowledge and information in a timely fashion to a major health services policy area is also seen in the development of hospices. Here the efforts of local entities persuaded Congress to make hospice services part of Medicare before HCFA could provide Congress with information from its recently implemented hospice demonstration projects. It appears that HCFA is better suited to play the role of a funding source than that of a primary provider of information.

CONCEPTUALIZING COMMUNITY-BASED LONG-TERM CARE: KINSTITUTION

Traditionally, care of the dependent—regardless of age—has been provided by more or less benign individuals in family groups, particularly women, and is referred to as "informal support." Research into informal support indicates that time and again most care has been given by family and friends (Cantor, 1979; Clark and Pelham, 1982; Shanas, 1979a; Shanas, 1979b). More specifically, the world of informal support, like the world of the aged, is primarily a world of women. One need only walk the halls of any nursing home in any town or city anywhere in the United States to observe that growing very old and working to care for the very old is predominantly a female experience. Additionally, the editors' own research into informal support under the roofs of hospitals and nursing homes indicates that this pattern of caring continues in these institutional settings (Clark and Pelham, 1982; Clark and Pelham, 1983). Significant amounts of work are undertaken and provided—often on a daily basis—for inpatients, even though paid staff persons may be numerous.

The predominance of this pattern will probably continue, but contemporary complexities have begun to overwhelm the caregivers of the very frail. The emotional, physical, and resource burdens placed upon loving people are increasing. What price are caregivers paying for these sacrifices? What are the hidden societal costs (e.g., divorce, stress-related illnesses, or elder abuse) of assuming these caring tasks? Love may be free, but loving for the long term can be an expensive proposition. In addition to these questions, others have been raised concerning the number of caregivers who will be available in the future as our population grows older and more numerous.

Community-based long-term care is a societal attempt to rally and focus technology, expertise, and resources to maintain the health, life, and independence of a needy elder whose natural systems have become worn or failed. In one sense, the notion of community-based long-term care is an attempt to duplicate the nature of the caring family—or more specifically, the caring wife or daughter. It attempts to create an institutional structure that functions like a surrogate family for its needy elder members.

The process of community-based long-term care developing

into a kind of family is extremely difficult, but the concept itself is not new. The Schatzman concept of "kinstitution" is especially useful for explaining this phenomenon (1982). A kinstitution is a hybrid, symbiotic relationship consisting of familial and formal organizational structures that serve to meet the needs of a particular individual or group.

One can conceptualize the "kin" component as the practice side of the dichotomy and the "institution" component as the organizational side. But this hybrid structure often creates an operational and functional schizophrenia for workers. While one is attempting to behave like a caring family member and provide services there are the distractions of paperwork and travel time. Additionally, there are the "transaction costs" of meetings and negotiating for services.

"Schizophrenia" for workers also results from the dissonance of attempting to reconcile conflicting and contradictory values. How can an advocate struggle to maintain an elder's personal autonomy while at the same time advising that the elder on Medicare reject his or her lifetime value system and "spend down"? In other words, the person is advised to become poor on purpose in order to become a welfare and Medicaid recipient who can receive supportive services at home that he or she could not afford to pay for out of pocket.

Metamorphosis of an institution into a kinstitution relationship and role is not unlike evolving into a caring daughter or son, husband or wife. Even given this formidable task, states across the nation and provinces in Canada have embarked upon major social experiments. By creating social and health services organizations to supplement and help coordinate informal support, agencies are creating kinstitutions to care for the needy aged at home.

PRESENT PRACTICE AND ORGANIZATIONAL ISSUES

This volume presents some of the issues, both practice and organizational, that have emerged in the field of community-based long-term care for the elderly. As more and more states become involved with this approach, the lessons learned will become more valuable. Specific articles in this volume come from the experiences of community-based long-term care research and demonstration projects funded by the Health Care Financing Administration (HCFA). Also included is a description of a Canadian initiative in this area. All contributors address different dimensions of caring for the frail, and often ill, aged at home through a case management approach with the provision of additional needed services. This appears on the surface to be a relatively straightforward notion. It is not.

Contributors of the following chapters illustrate and explain trial and error, joys and frustrations, and on-the-job expertise acquired by managing a community long-term care service agency. These stories are practical examples of contemporary applied gerontology.

Dennis Stone begins by opening the door to the examining room and offering a physician's advice concerning more effective physical and psychosocial care at home. Dr. Stone learned tricks of the trade of caring for the impaired elderly, who were often without families, in San Francisco's Tenderloin. He served as an innovative Medical Director of North of Market Senior Center for ten years. He points out that through the use of multidisciplinary staff and simple technology, impaired elders may remain autonomous in the community.

Browdie and Turwoski point out that being a kinstitution is not easy. They raise the practical, organizational issues involved in the logistics of providing services to the elderly in the community. They also describe how to work with the troubled and troublesome client. Any caregiving spouse or child will recognize these stories. They close their chapter with practical ideas for dynamic roles that workers may adopt for negotiating with and conquering multiple bureaucracies.

Kirby Shoaf, from Milwaukee, outlines the "paper trail" required of a kinstitution. Documents along the way include screening and assessment instruments, service plans and orders, and progress notes. Because community-based long-term care agencies often start out as research and demonstration projects, there is the parallel and intersecting paper trail of control groups, instrumentation, evaluations, and reports. Like any good pathfinder, he points out the pitfalls and shortcuts for those who are new to community-based long-term care.

Peters offers strategies for case managers to successfully intervene in one of the most critical episodes of an elder's life—hospitalization. The "ten commandments" instruct case managers how to imitate the behavior of an adept, caring family (e.g., to become a vigilant patient advocate). The orientation is toward client autonomy and a return home.

Betty Havens provides an international perspective on community-based long-term care by showing how Canadians in Manitoba successfully cross social service, health, and multiple private and public sector boundaries. She points out that so called "maverick" community-based social and health service agencies are unique in their ability to cross over and integrate disparate systems and to create systemic change. Lastly, she explores the boundary issues and challenges of the future.

Quinn and Rieck analyze high technology computer systems and applications currently in use in a New England community care agency. In many ways, the computer is the "nervous system" of a kinstitution. It recalls the tasks of creating the agency "brain," developing systems, inputting, short and long-term memory, and educating the agency "brain" and "body" to work together. They also acknowledge that "hardware" can be interpreted in more than one way!

Zlotnick and Weinstein present another perspective on the critical episode of hospitalization. They describe the organizational struggle of a community-based agency to "crack" hospitals in New York and bring home patients already assigned to nursing homes.

In "Interviewing Challenges," we explain the nature of the alien experience of interviewing poor, and often frail, ill elders in California. The California Senior Survey (CSS) served as the control group for the statewide Multipurpose Senior Services Project (MSSP). Elders were assessed on six-month schedules for three years in three subsamples drawn from the community, hospitals, and nursing homes. The realities of conducting survey research with this unique population are described in detail. We outline the "dos" and "don'ts" for panel studies and give the reader a concise recipe and "how to" instructions. Although they are sometimes embarrassing, we acknowledge that false starts, confusion, regroupings, errors, surprises, and humor are inherent in human attempts to study and help each other.

Weinstein and Zlotnick tackle perhaps the most delicate and emotionally charged dilemma of research and demonstration community-based long-term care: project termination. They show that, even given significant amounts of time for planning, anticipation of worst-case scenarios, and buying more time for a reprieve, the trauma of project termination was enormous. Suffering occurred on both sides of the desk—for clients and staff alike. The whole process is not unlike a family breakup with the care providers no longer there. They offer knowledge about how to mitigate this trauma and end with a plea for longer lives for human service demonstration projects.

Our final chapter grapples with projections into possible policy futures. We explore the relativistic nature and social construction of "the problem" of long-term care. We examine conflicting interests and ends of social actors involved in the long-term care wars. Finally, we take a stand for one single human value: personal autonomy. We then analyze and evaluate proposed social policy alternatives based upon our stated criteria. We conclude that the most feasible and probable policy option is an expansion of community-based long-term care. However, a national income policy, cashing out existing services, is our personal preference for the long-term future.

Since the field of community-based long-term care is relatively new, we have included some suggested materials in a bibliography for the reader who wishes to pursue further the topics discussed in this volume. The bibliography follows the references to this introduction.

REFERENCES

Cantor, M. H. Neighbors and friends. *Research on Aging*, 1979, *1*, 434-463.

Clark, W. F., & Pelham, A. O. *Who's taking care of the poor old widows now?* Paper presented at the 1982 Annual Meeting of the Midwest Sociological Society, Des Moines, Iowa, 1982.

Clark, W. F., & Pelham, A. O. *Informal support provided to a recent admissions cohort of Medicaid skilled nursing facility patients.* Paper presented at the Thirty-Sixth Annual Meeting of the Gerontological Society of America, San Francisco, Calif., 1983.

Kart, C. S., & Manard, B. B. Introduction. In C. S. Kart & B. B. Manard (Eds.), *Aging in America: Readings in social gerontology.* Sherman Oaks, Calif.: Alfred Publishing Co., 1976.

Katz, S., et al. *Effects of continued care.* Washington, D.C.: DHEW Publ. No. 73-3010, 1972.

Pelham, A. O., & Clark, W. F. *When do you go home: Hospital discharge and placement decisions for the elderly and implications for community-based long-term care agencies.* Paper presented at the Thirty-Fifth Annual Meeting of the Gerontological Society of America, Boston, Mass., 1982.

Schatzman, L. Professor of Sociology, University of California at San Francisco. Personal Communication, 1982.

Shanas, E. The family as a social support system in old age. *The Gerontologist*, 1979a, *19*, 169-174.

Shanas, E. Social myths as hypothesis: The case of the family relations of old people. *The Gerontologist*, 1979b, *19*, 3-9.

SUGGESTED READINGS

Specific Projects

Berkeley Planning Associates. *Evaluation of coordinated community-oriented long-term care demonstration projects, draft executive summary.* Berkeley, Calif.: Mimeo, 1984.

Katz, S., et al. *Effects of continued care.* Washington, D.C.: DHEW Publ. No. 73-3010, 1972.

Miller, L. S., Clark, M. L., & Clark, W. F. The comparative evaluation of California's Multipurpose Senior Services Project. *Home Health Care Quarterly Review*, in press.

Quinn, J., et al. *Coordinating community services for the elderly: The Triage experience.* New York, N.Y.: Springer Publishing Co., 1982.

Seidle, F. W., et al. *Delivering in-home services to the aged and disabled.* Lexington, Mass.: Lexington Books, 1983.

Skellie, A. F., Mobley, G. M., & Coan, R. E. Cost-effectiveness of community-based long-term care: Current findings of Georgia's Alternative Health Services Project. *American Journal of Public Health*, 1982, *72*, 353-358.

Thompson, E. *Home Care Program in Manitoba.* Paper presented at Prevention and Social Policy Conference of the Social Planning Council of Winnipeg and the Canadian Council on Social Development, Winnipeg, Canada, 1979.

Weissert, W. G., Wan, T. T. H., & Liveratos, B. B. *Effects and costs of day care and homemaker services for the chronically ill: A randomized experiment.* Hyattsville, Md.: National Center for Health Services Research, (PHS) 79-3250, 1979.

Zawadski, R. T. (Ed.) Community-based systems of long-term care. *Home Health Care Services Quarterly*, 1983, *4*.

Practice

Bennett, R., Frisch, S., Gurland, B., & Wilder, D. (Eds.) *Coordinated service delivery systems for the elderly: New approaches for care & referral in New York State.* New York, N.Y.: Haworth Press, 1984.

Burnside, I. M. *Nursing and the aged*, 2nd Ed. New York, N.Y.: McGraw-Hill, 1981.

Koff, T. H. *Long-term care: An approach to serving the frail elderly.* Boston, Mass.: Little, Brown and Co., 1982.
Rossman, I. (Ed.) *Clinical Geriatrics.* Philadelphia, Penn.: Lippincott Press, 1971.
Sheehan, S. *Kate Quinton's days.* Boston, Mass.: Houghton Mifflin Co., 1984.
Steinberg, R. M., & Carter, G. W. *Case management and the elderly.* Lexington, Mass.: Lexington Books, 1983.

Background

Estes, C. L., et al. *Fiscal austerity and aging: Shifting government responsibility for the elderly.* Beverly Hills, Calif.: Sage Publishing Co., 1983.
Federal Council on Aging. *Public policies and the frail elderly.* Washington, D.C.: U.S. Department of Health, Education, and Welfare, 1978.
Harrington, C., Newcomer, R. J., Estes, C. L., & associates. *Long term care of the elderly.* Beverly Hills, Calif.: Sage Publications, 1984.

Policy Studies

American Public Health Association. Toward a national policy on long-term care for the aging. *American Journal of Public Health,* 1982, *72,* 207-210.
Callahan, J. J., Jr., & Wallack, S. S. (Eds.) *Reforming the long-term care system.* Lexington, Mass.: Lexington Books, 1981.
Congressional Budget Office. *Long-term care for the elderly and disabled: Budget issue paper.* Washington, D.C.: U.S. Government Printing Office, 1979.
Doherty, N., Segal, J., & Hicks, B. Alternatives to institutionalization for the aged: Viability and cost effectiveness, a review of the literature. *Aged Care & Services Review,* 1978, *1,* 1-16.
Dunlop, B. D. Expanded home-based care for the elderly: Solution or pipe dream? *American Journal of Public Health,* 1980, *70,* 514-519.
Eustis, N., Greenberg, J., & Patten, S. *Long-term care for older persons: A policy perspective.* Monterey, Calif.: Brooks-Cole Publishing Co., 1984.
Kane, R. L., & Kane, R. A. *A will and a way: What the United States can learn from Canada about care of the elderly.* New York: Columbia University Press, 1985.
U.S. General Accounting Office. *The elderly should benefit from expanded home care but increasing these services will not insure cost reductions.* Washington, D.C.: U.S. General Accounting Office, 1982.

Nursing Homes

Vladeck, B. C. *Unloving care.* New York, N.Y.: Basic Books, 1980.

1

Maintaining and Improving the Functional Status of the Frail Elderly

Dennis Stone

INTRODUCTION

Millions of elders in this country have some impairment in their ability to perform the basic activities of daily life. This affects not only the elders themselves, but more importantly, their spouses, their children, other relatives, neighbors, and friends. The basic American ethics of family, self-determination, independence, and self-reliance are so intertwined that elders may not expect or realize the amount of energy that is really going into the maintenance of their life at home. That energy, unfortunately, is finite. If it is overtaxed, the elder may have no alternative but institutional placement. There are, however, many things that can be done to make sure that this energy is used efficiently.

Often, the elder wishes to "go it alone, no matter what." Even in such cases, help is possible through the introduction of new skills and tools. In other cases, care providers—whether family, friends, or professionals—are involved. The problems with providing such care, no matter how difficult, are not unique. Many "tricks of the trade" exist that can help maintain the independence of the frail elder.

POSTHOSPITALIZATION HOME CARE

Although chronic disease is the primary factor that decreases functioning in the elderly, it is often the period shortly after discharge from institutional care that is the most critical time in the elder's readjustment to independent living. We often think of the term "rehabilitation" as something that only takes place after a stroke, a fracture, or a traumatic episode. Unfortunately, professional care providers also often think in these terms, too. Equally incorrect is the thought that rehabilitation can only take place in an institutional setting. The World Health Organization defines rehabilitation as "the combined and coordinated use of medical, social, educational, and vocational measures for training and retraining the individual to the highest possible level of functional ability." This is far from just a short run through a rehabilitation program prior to release from a hospital. Even this definition, however, leaves out one important factor: emotional outlook. It is this outlook above all that helps maintain the elder's determination and the helper's stamina. It must be remembered by those involved that they need not feel alone—help in many forms is available.

As Director of Services for ten years in a community-based long-term care program in San Francisco's Tenderloin district, I have seen even the best discharge plans fall apart for many reasons. The most frequent problems were miscommunication, incomplete assessment, and poor follow-up. The physician, as primary prescriber of health care, previously acted as "gatekeeper" of all professional in-home support services. In today's world of health delivery, however, much has to be assessed and implemented outside the traditional axis of hospital–nursing home–doctor's office. What happens in the home is really what determines how often the elder needs to enter a physician's care. Little knowledge of that home ever reaches the physician unless he or she takes the time for family conferences, case conferences, or house calls.

All too often I would see an elder who was discharged home on Friday (traditional hospital house-cleaning day) return to the same milieu that precipitated the initial hospitalization. A return to such things as:

- a walk-up apartment left as it was the night the elder was taken to the hospital;
- an unmade bed, empty refrigerator, and signs of incontinence or vomitus;
- a complicated schedule of medications, with the risk of either under or over-medication;
- an elderly spouse suffering from his or her own chronic disorders; and

- an uninformed family, neighbor, or hotel manager who has not the slightest idea what the elder's sickness was in the first place, or what to do for the elder now.

In a more sophisticated health delivery system, long before discharge, many disciplines work to prepare the elder for transition back to functional independence. Physicians are busy fine-tuning the healing process. Nurses administer care and supportive environments needed to regain full health. Multiple therapists provide initial mechanisms for regaining specialized skills. Social workers arrange for psychosocial and financial tools that will be needed for the elder's return to the home environment. There needs to be intensive communication among all these disciplines and with the elder and any other supportive parties if the transition is to be smooth and successful. Communication and care cannot, however, stop at the threshold of the institution. It must be facilitated, perhaps indefinitely, through some agent such as the social worker, the public health nurse, a case manager, or a family member. The physician may continue to play a gatekeeper role in this ongoing care, but now he or she must play the role in a team context.

The role of the natural support system of family, friends, church, and neighbors should never be forgotten by the professional system. Despite the profound family neglect of elders I saw in the Tenderloin, most American families willingly accept their role as care providers (but often without any skills to help them in that role).What is determined by the professional's thorough assessment and therapy needs to be carefully communicated and negotiated with the elder and those involved at home. Often this information is transmitted at a time when the elder is still quite ill or debilitated, or when families are too intimidated to really hear what is being said. It is important, therefore, that a written "treatment plan" be available so that it can be carefully read later when it may be more clearly understood. It will also have to be periodically updated as functional status changes either for the better or the worse.

DISABILITIES AND LIVING AT HOME

We will now look at some suggestions to help counteract some of the major disabilities that may limit a frail elder's function and independence while living at home.

Ambulation

Loss of ambulation can vary from having a massive stroke to "just not being able to get about like I used to." Limitations can result from loss of motor control, pain, or limitation of joint function. Motivation also plays a very important role in any of these factors. Use of ambulation devices, including crutches, walkers, and canes, are often assessed as needed and prescribed while the patient is hospitalized for an acute episode. The situation and need for such appliances changes instantly when elders return home. Gone are the tiled uniform floors of the hospital. Gone is the person who can always put the appliance in the correct position before transfer. It is interesting how often these appliances are replaced at home with doorknobs, chair backs, and walls as mechanisms of support as the elders get about. Pride often has something to do with the refusal to use the device, but often the reason is the environment itself. Wheelchairs just do not work on soft carpet. Walkers do not help much getting across an area rug. Canes seem always to be on the other side of the room.

Expensive wall-mounted railings may be installed as an excellent aid to ambulation. Perhaps the best method is to help the elder rearrange the furniture in such a way that it does, indeed, act as an ambulation support. Walls are not half bad as a stabilizing factor. A fall by sliding down along a wall is often less traumatic than a fall over one's walker. A physical therapist or occupational therapist's in-home assessment can often be the key for putting such a system in order. Other specifics to consider are remembering to:

- remove as many area rugs as the elder will permit;
- remove as many small tables and other low lying obstacles as the elder will allow. However, these tables are often filled with knickknacks and photos of an elder's cherished world, and it is difficult to redistribute them in a home already filled with memories;
- make sure all pathways through the house are illuminated, either with activating wall switches or bright nightlights. They now make beeper and voice-activated wall outlets that can turn on lights remotely while the elder is still in bed or at the threshold of a room;
- make sure any ambulation device can get through a door jam. Often the problem is a matter of an inch or two

which can be resolved simply by taking the door off the hinges. The bathroom door can be replaced with a shower curtain;

- think about closing off the upstairs and moving the sleeping room downstairs. *Stairs are always trouble*;
- keep in mind that ramps, often thought to be the answer to an outside stair problem, can get slippery with rain or mold. Even in "sunny California," sidewalks and stepping stones may be slippery in winter months. Think about adhesive strips with nonskid surfaces applied to these areas (available at boating stores);
- think about footwear. It needs to be nonskid, soled, comfortable, and easy to get on and off. If you find a good pair, go back and buy two or three more, as you may never find them again;
- support impaired joints, thus reducing the stress that can produce pain. Athletes often use special joint wraps for knees and ankles which older people could also use. These are easier to put on than Ace bandages and are available at most sports stores. They should not be used by elders with circulatory problems or for extended periods of time;
- consider that the height of chairs and beds often makes simple acts of getting up and down precarious. Raising them may be beneficial, but make sure that the elder gets used to the new height, thereby averting falls in the middle of the night. Also avoid swivel chairs—in which accidents can easily happen;
- never forget foot care. At our Senior Clinic, if there was ever an argument in the waiting room, it was over who got to see the podiatrist first. Elders living alone are often prone to poor foot care because of loss of needed dexterity or simple neglect. The results can be infection or a fall causing permanent and probably preventable damage;
- consider a wheelchair as a boon or a bane. Inappropriate use can allow an elder an easy way out of an ambulation problem. This short-term relief can, however, lead to permanent confinement with eventual sores on the buttocks or the tightening of the knee joints into a permanent flexed position known as a contracture. Once when I was evaluating an elder's skill in transferring from wheelchair to bed, I asked her to make the transfer. Forgetting to lock

her braces, she started up. I gently restrained her effort and said, "No, you forgot to do something first. What is the very first thing you must do before ever getting out of a wheelchair?" She paused for a moment. Then, with a sparkle in her eye, proclaimed, "Say, 'Mother may I?' ";

- use a seat belt as an excellent safety device for a wheelchair as well as the car; and,
- keep in mind that elders or their families often express fear that there may be a fall when the elder is left alone. They fear that many hours may go by before someone responds to the unheard calls for help. Sadly, this fear has led many elders to give up their homes and move to a nursing facility. With today's technology, this does not have to happen. "Lifeline" and many other companies now offer table model and wristband emergency devices that will automatically call a 24-hour monitored center when activated. These devices can allow two-way conversation, dispatch of an ambulance, or a call to the family for minor help. They may also provide regular "check-in times" to give elders a feeling of security.

Incontinence

Often the final straw, the development of incontinence can be the reason elders or families give up and opt for an institutional facility. Any person who develops this problem deserves an intensive medical evaluation. The statement, "Well, what do you expect, the patient is getting old," is not acceptable. No other reason, excluding dementia, causes more permanent institutional placement. If, after such a work-up, it is evident that even with medication or surgery the problem will continue, there are several methods to minimize the problem. Let us look at the types of incontinence and how to address their care.

Urinary Stress Incontinence. Urinary stress incontinence is caused by weakness of pelvic muscles that control bladder emptying. It is associated with sudden moves, coughing, bearing down, or laughing. It is made worse by diuretics (water pills for heart failure or high blood pressure). To reduce the consequences of the problem:

- avoid tight fitting clothes (e.g., girdles or belts);
- wear specially designed underwear with compartments for disposable absorbent pads;
- make frequent trips to the bathroom to "lighten the load";
- have a bedside commode or urinal handy; and
- plan your outings with several stops prearranged.

Urinary Overflow Incontinence. Urinary overflow incontinence is caused by the bladder not responding correctly to the accumulation of urine until it is overfilled and then released dramatically. This is seen in elders with a neurological rather than a muscle control problem. Besides considering the above precautions:

- ask your physician or physical therapist how to manipulate the bladder to allow for maximal emptying when urinating. This can be done by applying external pressure to the bladder;
- rethink use of a permanent catheter when suggested by the elder or the family. This is usually only used as a last resort because of the very likely danger of frequent urinary infections;
- reconsider the use of plastic coverings for chairs and beds. Be careful of placing plastic sheets on the floor (they can be tripped over) or on the bed under the sheet (they may encourage a bedsore if not properly supported); and,
- time your liquid intake so that you are not asking for trouble by drinking a lot of fluid before going out or to bed. Remember, however, that dehydration is a common cause of falls, constipation, fainting, and even hospitalization. Do not restrict fluids too much. Occasional incontinence is cheaper than a hospital stay.

Fecal Incontinence. Fecal incontinence is a major burden to all involved. This may be due to the loss either of conscious, muscle, or neurological control. It may even be due to impaction with resultant overflow around the blocked rectum. Again, a thorough work-up is required and may provide clues for treatment including:

- balancing diet and bulk to keep the stool on the firm side and then evacuating the bowel periodically with stimulant laxatives or enemas. A consultation with a dietitian or a public health nurse can be very valuable when using this method;
- scheduling bowel movements. As with urinary incontinence, timing may be all-important. The gastrocolic reflex occurs when something enters the stomach, causing stimulation for the emptying of the bowel. Simply trying to go to the bathroom after a meal often gets excellent results;
- arranging frequent and good hygiene for the bedbound patient. This can often mean the difference between bedsores and comfort. With any form of incontinence, this is a vital issue and arrangements must be made for this kind of care. When all family members are employed and out of the house, this can lead to institutionalization unless aide services can be procured. Consultation with a social worker or a case manager may help;
- using a bedpan if the patient is still alert and aware of the urge to go. Bedpans, especially a "fracture pan," may be the answer when no one is around. This, however, requires dexterity not always present in elderly patients. A therapist may be able to help the elder develop these skills;
- having a bell or call buzzer at the bedside can often avoid unnecessary accidents, but a quick response is a necessity because the time between urge and incontinence may be very short. A call buzzer in the bathroom is also important for an often neglected physiological fact. When an elder bears down at stool, it can affect blood pressure and heart rate and, in rare incidences, precipitate a fainting episode. Having a buzzer or support side rails by the toilet may prevent a major accident; and,
- providing clear and easy access to the bathroom. If elders are able to ambulate to the bathroom, make sure the room is always lighted, clothes are easily removable, and the toilet seat is raised for easy use.

All of these things may help cut down the time to a point where accidents will be fewer and farther between.

ENVIRONMENTAL INTERACTION

Environmental interactive problems can include loss of cognitive skills (understanding and memory), psychological, sight, hearing, or speech problems. They also include problems revolving around bathing and the sexual life. Finally, there is the special case of the bedbound elder. They can be the cause of great frustration both for elders and for those who care for them. Glasses and hearing aids are often not worn for various reasons including discomfort and the feeling that they "don't help," "don't work," or "make the problem worse." All these complaints may be true. What we discuss here goes beyond making sure that the appliances are appropriate and operating. There are a lot of answers but none are right for all cases. They may, however, help improve the quality of life for some of those afflicted. Remember, we are "trying to add life to years, not just years to life."

Cognition (Understanding and Memory)

Typical of this problem are Alzheimer's patients. Locked into an ever downward spiral of loss of ability to be functionally aware of one's own environment, this problem is exceptionally difficult for care providers. Included in ways to cope with this problem should be:

- having the patience of a saint;
- learning skills in reality therapy—frequent verbal cueing of time, place, names of family, and reminders of appropriate behavior;
- using visual clues of the past to keep the environment as familiar as possible (e.g., family pictures, knickknacks, or family furniture);
- scheduling of regular activities including eating, bathing, toileting, sleeping, physical activities, and "quality time" for intensive one-on-one interchanges;
- scheduling of concurrent mental health breaks for all care persons involved to prevent burnout. Use of respite care, adult day health centers, and senior center activities can often mean the difference between functioning at home and nursing home placement;

- being aware of "sundowning," that critical period of the day when fatigue and changing illumination start to distort already marginal functional skills;
- consulting with a physician skilled in these problems to make sure there is not a medically reversible cause for the behavior problem and to see if appropriate medication may be used to help modify particularly disruptive behavior;
- setting limits between elders and their caregivers to keep guilt from becoming an overriding factor in a caring relationship. It is all right to get frustrated and angry when dealing with this problem—it is normal. If resentment is allowed to grow, a crisis may develop later that will be regretted; and,
- sharing the work. Do not try to go it alone, it will only shorten the period before burnout sets in. Professional help often means the difference.

Psychological

Besides problems of dementia or cognitive impairment, one must also deal with basic psychosocial considerations. These may include loss of spouse (the death rate of the surviving spouse is 50 percent higher the year after such a loss), loneliness, organic depression, other forms of psychiatric illness, and sexual expression. None of these is easily handled by the elder alone. Help from the natural support system and counseling from professionals may improve attitude and thus, function.

Medicine has taken great steps forward since the days when tranquilizers were the only form of treatment available. True organic depression can be significantly reversed with medications now available. Support groups, each focusing on specific disabilities, are now available in many communities to help elders and those who care for them. These may include Stroke Groups, Cardiac Rehabilitation Groups, Post-Mastectomy Groups, or Associations of Alzheimer's and Related Disorders. A social worker or the local Office on Aging will help locate such groups in your area.

Use of senior centers, friendly visitor programs, or telephone reassurance services opens new roles and supports to previously isolated elders. This can be a vital means of changing those all important attitudes and rekindling the drive to live independently.

These activities also open the elder to "peer counseling" and he or she may find that their condition is not all that bad after all. Nothing is a better teacher than experience. Many valuable lessons can be picked up by being in contact with others who have already faced some of the problems of functional loss.

Sight

Usually loss of sight is a gradual process in elders. Along the way, special aids can be added to help maintain function. Help may include:

- never changing the layout of furniture, utensils, kitchen, tools, or rugs (except to get rid of those pesky area rugs);
- providing large type books and talking books available through most libraries;
- avoiding back lighting when interacting with an elder because it is difficult to discern features in that kind light;
- coding articles with bright colors for easier identification;
- arranging medications in dispensing compartments to reduce confusion; and,
- having an occupational therapist visit the home for special skill-building techniques.

Hearing

Again, hearing loss is usually a gradual process and often not noticed until it is quite severe because the patient may become quite adept at lip reading without noticing that he or she is doing it. There are still many things that can help the elder:

- remembering that hearing aids make all sounds louder, so that ambient noise can be quite irritating. When conversing with an elder with or without a hearing aid, it is best to turn off the TV and have the kids go in the other room to play;
- using some of the many other aids to hearing that have been developed including hearing wands for use during direct communication. Telephone receiver amplifiers are also available through many telephone equipment suppliers;
- using letter boards may be a more rapid way of communicating with elders if the hearing impairment is severe;

- speaking clearly and distinctly, though not necessarily more loudly, and keeping the light toward your face, will facilitate lip reading; and,
- keeping the ears clean. Those hard of hearing also get wax in their ears, making marginal hearing even worse; so ask your physician to remove it periodically. (Remember the "Elbow Rule.")

Speech

This can be a problem because of loss of ability to form words or inability to remember the exact words to use. Careful evaluation has to be made to see if using a letter board, a picture set, signing, a keyboard and a video screen, or simply a paper and pencil is the most efficient means to communicate. There is somebody inside still trying to express all the natural wishes and feelings they have always had. Communication is vital if that person is ever to have an acceptable quality of life again. A speech therapist evaluation is absolutely necessary for anyone with a communication problem. Suggestions from that evaluation will make life significantly better for all involved.

Bathing

Joys of a good hot bath or shower should always be remembered in maintaining the frail elder's comfort and function. Many appliances have been produced to make this still feasible for those living at home. They are easily installed and can include:

- bathseats, both in-tub and transfer platforms extending from tubs out over the floor to slide across;
- hand held shower nozzles;
- grab rails to be affixed to the wall or clamped on to tubs;
- adhesive strips to be placed on floors and in tubs; and,
- soap on a rope may make things a lot easier for everyone.

Bathing of one's own parent can often be a delicate situation, whether it is in the tub or a bed bath. It is often a help to have an outside aide, at least at the start, to alleviate the initial awkwardness of the situation. Also, remember the trick nurses use in the hospital of providing a bath for all but the personal areas and then letting the elder finish up on his or her own if at all possible.

Sex

An often not discussed aspect of an elder's life, sex is frequently neglected because professionals and care providers are the ones who wish to avoid the issue. It still remains a personal thing but it is very important to many elders and certainly a valid means of psychosocial support. Things that need to be considered include:

- remembering that elders still have a sexual image of themselves. Loss of a spouse, a mastectomy or prostatectomy, or the present cultural focus on youth make it extremely difficult for an elder to think of him/herself as sexually desirable. Special interest in grooming, remembering her jewelry or his hat, or simply an occasional compliment may be that special boost in morale that can keep them going;
- keeping in mind that opportunities can also be stacked against the elder. A senior center is definitely not a singles bar, and courtship is still regulated by mores of fifty years ago. Privacy is all but lost when family or professional care providers are involved in so many aspects of the elder's life. It leaves little space for sexual activity. Private occasions must be considered and respected. A giggle or an offhand remark may destroy a very fragile arrangement. *Be tactful*;
- understanding that the ability to actually perform the sexual act is also often compromised by physical impairment. A man may feel under pressure to perform. The woman may fear discomfort from a dry vaginal area. Physicians may be able to help in many cases by being aware that many of the medications prescribed may be causing impotence as a side effect or that there are medications available to revitalize the vaginal canal;
- bearing in mind that consultation from peers, church, or professionals is more often sought than advice from family. Those honored with a request for advice should give it freely, nonjudgmentally, maturely, and with encouragement; and,
- always remembering how important sex and physical affection have been to you.

Bedbound

The problem of being bedbound, whether transient or chronic, can be a challenge to elders and those wishing to help. Dangers of further loss of function, contractures, bedsores, pneumonia, and boredom all have to be considered. A key to survival and, perhaps, reambulation is, again, attitude and determination on the part of all parties involved. Special consideration should be given to the following areas.

Exercise. Either passive or, preferably, active exercise must be scheduled frequently during the day to prevent any and all of the above consequences. Within two days of staying in bed, muscle strength starts to decline, and within one week, early contractures can be noted. There is definitely a danger in letting elders rest "comfortably" all day in bed. A simple act of moving each joint through its complete range of motion can, in the long run, determine whether the patient will live the rest of her or his life as someone up and about or someone contracted up into a grotesque ball with their heels in the buttocks and their arms twisted across their chest. Types of exercise should include:

- isotonic or active movement by elders themselves utilizing each muscle group. This can be taught by a physical therapist to those elders capable of doing this level of activity on their own. Isometrics are not encouraged because of dangers related to "bearing down" mentioned earlier; and,
- passive range of motion exercise can also be taught by the physical therapist to care providers of elders who cannot presently perform a particular exercise on their own.

Aids. Tools that can be included to prevent motor decline may include:

- an overhead trapeze to facilitate increased strength in shoulder muscles and also to allow for easier transfers or for changing the bed;
- a footboard to help prevent the gradual contracture of ankles caused by unopposed force of the strong Achilles' tendon. Without something to push against, the classic tiptoe deformity will develop; and,
- siderails to prevent inadvertent falling out of bed at night. Remember, however, that siderails are a leading cause of incontinence for the immobile bedbound.

Bedsores (Decubiti). A constant danger for bedbound elders, bedsores first appear as a slightly reddened area but can suddenly break down into draining, inflamed, large lesions that can take months to heal. They can also become sites of infection that can lead to more dangerous health problems. For prevention, consider:

- percale sheets or a sheepskin mattress pad which helps reduce the trauma of constant rubbing of the skin on the sheets;
- an eggshell mattress, a waterbed, or an air mattress to distribute the weight of bony prominences of hips, buttocks, sacrum, and heels;
- heel protectors or "space boots" to again prevent a sore in this particularly vulnerable spot. This is especially dangerous for elders with diabetes or peripheral vascular disease;
- frequent turning from side to back to side to alleviate pressure on any one area. Unrelieved pressure kills the tissue underneath. It is as if a tourniquet had been applied. Long periods on the stomach may be dangerous if the elder is prone to coughing or choking;
- absolute insistence on a clean, dry bed because chronic exposure to dampness easily breaks down the skin; and,
- a catheter is not the answer to all incontinence problems because it opens the way to infection. It should only be considered when healing existing decubiti (sores) depends on such vigorous techniques.

Pneumonia. An ever present danger for the bedbound elder, pneumonia develops because secretions tend to collect at the base of the lungs and allows bacteria to get a foothold. The best prevention technique is to get the elder up in a chair or at least sitting up in bed frequently during the day. In severely debilitated persons with chronic respiratory problems, there is a vast array of equipment available including respirators, suction devices, oxygen dispensers, atomizers, and intermittent breathing machines that can be utilized at home. A respirator therapist can be made available to train elders or care providers in their use, function, and maintenance.

Eating. The simple act of eating can be a real challenge to elders or to care providers in the bedbound situation or if motor or emotional problems are involved. However, specialized aids can make it a bit easier, including:

- compartmentalized dishes for patients with a motor problem or who are blind;
- nonskid plates and cups with expanded bases (both are available at boating stores) which prevent spills and the chasing of things all over the tray;
- attachable plate backstops to help the elder get the food on to utensils more easily (available at many medical supplies stores);
- swivel utensils to help elders with a tremor counteract the swaying motion of the hand (also available at a medical supplies store); and,
- the lowly straw for soup, custards, and diluted pureed meals.

Preparing the meal, itself, can be a challenge because of limitations of special diets. Also, the general layout of a kitchen can be trying if the elder with motor impairment is trying to still cook for him or herself. Special guidance from a dietitian or a home visit by an occupational therapist can help in many situations. Also, consider the use of a timer on a toaster oven or a microwave as a method of cooking rather than using a gas or electric stove. These stoves have the inherent danger of being left on or being reached across while the elder is wearing loose fitting garments.

Boredom. Besides those subjects and alternatives noted under emotional considerations, bedbound elders may have particular problems keeping mentally active. A visit by a recreational or occupational therapist may help with such suggestions as:

- mounting the TV from an elevated wall mount so elders having to lie flat can still see the program;
- remote hearing plugs so the TV does not disturb others and at the same time is more easily heard by the elder;
- a tiltable bed table so a book can be placed in a comfortable position for reading;
- multiple craft projects that can be done even while bedbound; and,
- for the very alert, political volunteer phone campaigning is always needed by candidates and can really keep the elder's self-esteem high since it is a very relevant activity.

SUMMARY

The functional range of the frail elder can run from totally capable in all aspects of physical and mental activity to the elder who can no longer manage any aspect of their activities of daily living. Using the natural support system and the multidisciplinary professional support available in one's community can add many years to functional independence. Providing access to that support can be very difficult given today's bureaucracy, health delivery systems, and professional rivalries. Once one knows what to expect, what to do, and who can help do it, things start to fall into place. A case manager may be of help in the more complicated cases, but it is usually still up to family members to at least start the process. Any care professional should be able to help you "access the system." Getting the system to communicate and coordinate is the name of the game.

I have had patients who have remained at home for many years—bedbound, confused, alone, or with family. The successful ones are those who keep their determination and who use many of the suggestions noted in this chapter.

2

The Problems of Providing Services to the Elderly in Their Own Homes

Richard Browdie and Adrian Turwoski

PROBLEMS IN THE LONG-TERM CARE SYSTEM

Long-term care currently suffers from a lack of clarity concerning the roles of the many organizations, practitioners, and levels of government involved. A worker in this field faces the prospect of contending with client needs, agency policies, referral and intake protocols, turf rivalries, and service gaps without any precise tools to engineer a workable care plan. The instability of many frail older persons' physical capacities, informal supports, and social environments means that a care plan must be a flexible and responsive collection of services. Needed services must come from paid and unpaid sources. The worker "sews" them together. To continue the sampler analogy, the system currently does not routinely provide financing for all of the "stitches" necessary, nor administrative "needles" to knit them as the worker encounters problems in the field.

What if all roles were sorted out? What if all gaps were filled, sufficient financing arranged, the "stitches" available in adequate supply and the "needles" distributed to those who might need them? Would this eliminate all difficulties in providing services to homebound elderly?

Of course not. This is because many problems that are encountered in delivering services to our homebound elderly arise from the very nature of the business. The two major problem areas that we will discuss are logistical types of problems and client-related problems. We end this chapter with a description of different roles one can adopt to cope with these problematic areas.

LOGISTICAL PROBLEMS

Location: Everywhere

To begin with, the clientele is not located in any single convenient place. This distribution problem gives rise to logistical problems that present a challenge to an individual worker, not to mention an agency supervisor or administrator. Simply getting to all clients as frequently and as quickly as necessary is a serious problem, particularly for workers in rural areas and in heavily congested urban areas. Face-to-face encounters are critically important if the worker is going to be able to knowledgeably assist a client in a decision-making process. It also may be the only opportunity to understand clearly what is going on with a client and his or her environment. If those client encounters, which themselves may take a significant amount of time, require large amounts of travel time to and between clients' homes, fewer visits can be made.

Travel constitutes a considerable obstacle for both workers and administrators. For the worker, travel time is a constant burden which occupies time and energy that could be better spent with clients or in finishing off that interminable paper work, part of which the travel itself generates for documentation and reimbursement purposes. Travel contributes to an already difficult job and can lead to faster case manager burnout. It can also be expensive for workers, because of only partially compensated wear and tear on personal automobiles and increased insurance expenses because of business use. In some communities, business-related use of a personally owned automobile can almost double the rate charged by insurance companies. Finally, statistical possibilities of becoming involved in an accident or having a breakdown go up considerably, along with the general stress of moving about in all sorts of weather.

For administrators and supervisors, travel needs are a thorny problem as well. The most obvious problem is productivity. Long travel times lead to lower productivity and/or higher costs. Fewer cases can be seen in a day, paper work and recording is delayed, demand for reimbursement of expenses goes up and supervisory controls are stretched. In some contexts, workers may need to be contacted on short notice while they are out in the field. Long travel periods obviously make that more difficult.

Normal case work supervisory functions are more difficult as well. Scheduling supervisory visits with workers and clients becomes difficult and scheduling office conferences can be a problem because of the perception that all time available has to be spent in the field with needy clients. There also is a constant pressure to balance workers' time between clients and paper work because of the temptation to take the easy way out and only go into the field on rare occasions—thereby avoiding hassles. This leads, naturally, to a drop in quality of information that caseworkers have available to them and, therefore, threatens the quality of their decision making and practice. It can also lead to mistakes which are injurious to clients and their interests, to disgruntled family members, and to disenchanted politicians and others in authority. The environment of a frail elderly client is a complex web of interacting elements. Misunderstanding a change in one element, because of a lack of contact with the client, can result in an unanticipated but preventable crisis. Family members, who may or may not have been involved, will frequently "go to the source," which often is perceived as being a political figure, or a chief administrator, or both. Some situations like this will happen even when the worker is on top of things. But if the worker missed something that he or she would have noticed had they seen their client, the potential for trouble is obvious.

From an administrator's point of view, travel and productivity are countervailing factors in underwriting costs of services. More caseworkers are needed if travel consumes an inordinate amount of time and money. Conversely, fewer clients can be served and waiting lists get longer. If resources are being allocated to competing program needs from a single source, then geographic characteristics of areas served are significant factors in determining just how much money can be invested in service management functions.

This same sort of problem affects costs and responsiveness of other services as well. Greater travel demands means a more expensive and less productive care-giving work force. For higher paid personnel, the problem is greater. But there are two other related problems that deserve special attention: quality of care and service coordination.

Quality of Care Logistics

The first problem is that of assuring quality of care. It is a fact of life that people must be held accountable if the quality of their work is to be assured. A process of assuring quality care is extremely difficult from the perspectives both of case managers and of service providers. Case managers find it very difficult to be on site to witness service provision because of difficulties getting to the homes of multiple clients, each of whom may be receiving several services on the same days. Providers find supervisory problems described for service managers are multiplied for their own workers.

In the first place, service providers have a function which is more hands-on than administrative. This means that supervisors have to be with a staff person to witness what is going on. A case plan review will not tell them anything, and clients themselves are often not reliable informants. An impaired elder may be afraid to "tell" on a lazy homemaker for fear of losing service or incurring the homemaker's wrath. The client may also have cognitive impairments that do not permit them to perceive good or bad performance and/or to accurately relate their observations to others. Provider agencies typically also have relatively high staff to supervisor ratios. Each staff person has multiple clients in scattered locations and faces a wide variety of circumstances. A supervisor has quite a challenge assuring high quality in their subordinates' work.

From a provider's point of view, costs of assuring quality can be a real problem in addition to the logistical difficulties described. Providers are often paid a fixed fee for each unit of service provision, normally in the form of a per visit, per hour, or other unit cost reimbursement. Costs of supervision and quality assurance must be taken out of that fixed payment, and even the sharpest negotiators have difficulty passing all of those costs back to payers, particularly if competitive bidding practices are used. In today's service system, more and more firms providing care to our homebound are profit-making firms. Many of them are owned by national companies. A local office manager, small businessperson, or franchise operator must make a profit if they are to survive. No matter how well intentioned they are or how high their ethical standards are, even a nonprofit provider has an incentive to cut costs on internal procedures for quality assurance and shift to a pattern where problems are addressed after they occur. This is a natural and understandable temptation. However, it leads to a reduction in the consistency of an agency's demand for its workers to do high quality work. Unfortunately, that will usually lead to reduced quality of care for long-term care clients.

Service Coordination Logistical Problems with Other Staff

Case conferences present another major problem caused by logistical difficulties intrinsic to community care concerns and coordination functions. Coordination of services, after all, is one of the major goals of service management. One of the most popular and effective means of coordinating the activities of a number of actors on behalf of one client is to have a case conference. Yet case conferences can be logistically very difficult to put together when providers are scattered about. Conferences with providers of care can also be expensive, because time spent in conferences is lost to providers who would otherwise be earning reimbursements. Logically, providers are reluctant to permit their personnel to go to such meetings unless they are paid. If they are paid, it is an expense incurred that produces no direct care, which makes administrators reluctant to pay for such events with any frequency.

Service Coordination Logistical Problems with Families

Coordination is one of the primary objectives of service management. It is a problem that must be addressed if clients' needs are to be effectively met. But a related problem that may be even more crucial in home care of the elderly is coordination with and support of the families of older persons. It is now a widely known fact that families and friends, known collectively as informal caregivers, provide the majority of care for older persons. Those with experience in managing care for very frail elders at home learn that the willingness and ability of informal caregivers to be involved is crucial. Informal caregivers can make the difference between providing cost effective community-based care and care at home which is prohibitively expensive. Therefore, maintenance and nurturing of informal supports and coordination of activities of formal services providers with informal caregivers are probably the most critical coordinating functions of service managers.

Though each family and network of informal support differs, they commonly need a certain amount of counseling and attention as they strive to care for their loved one in often tremendously difficult circumstances. This "care and feeding" function requires building and maintenance of relationships, which in turn requires face-to-face encounters with some regularity. Scattered locations again mitigate against carrying out this function. But of all problems, this is the one that a service manager, indeed the whole service management system, can least afford to ignore. Family and friends are foundations upon which a system of care for the homebound elderly must be built. A failure to acknowledge this and to plan for it in development of a long-term care system, from an individual case plan to an area-wide system, will certainly lead to failure in many cases where success could be attained.

CLIENT RELATED PROBLEMS

Reliability

One of the most fundamental issues that must be addressed in designing community-based long-term care systems is how to interact appropriately with clients and families. A worker and his or her supervisor are faced with negotiating with families and clients around what they will do versus what formal care can be provided. In the majority of cases, informal caregivers are reliable and durable. They can be counted on. When not so, they make the case planning process tremendously difficult because of the instability that they induce. To deal with unreliable informal supports, a worker must arrange for extra services and/or constantly adjust care plans to accommodate short-range changes in the conduct of unpaid caregivers. Possibilities for confusion with and among formal service providers can be a severe problem as well. In most cases, tasks that formal service providers are assigned are designed to complement what the family and friends can do, and if the behavior and availability of familial supports are unreliable, task assignments are thrown into chaos, particularly if multiple providers are involved.

Implications of problematic informal support for caseworkers and their organizations are obvious. Coordination time and costs climb dramatically. Clients whose physical conditions are cause for day-to-day concern are unstable enough. An unreliable family compounds problems and may quickly lead to an elder's institutionalization. Costs of care brought in to assure the client's safety in lieu of reliable informal support becomes prohibitively expensive. Less dangerous to the client, but as problematic for workers, is the relatively high incidence of angry formal service providers in a situation of unstable informal supports. Service personnel frequently feel that they have enough trouble getting to a client's home and performing a service in less than ideal circumstances with severe time and cost constraints. An unpredictable family member can quickly become the proverbial "last straw." This sort of situation creates huge problems for caseworkers, and may lead to an unraveling of a whole plan of care, thereby threatening a client's well-being.

Informational Problems and the Family

A second problem area relating to informal supports is one that should not be terribly difficult to manage, but which can lead to serious difficulties—that is, information. From the moment a worker makes contact with a client and their informal supports, they begin to collect information from them. The focus of most of these data is the client, their level of functioning, unmet needs, and continuing welfare after a plan of care has been implemented. The flow of accurate information is crucial to the worker's interpretation of needs and resources and, therefore, the accuracy and efficacy of assessment decisions and care plans.

Problems begin with the fact that clients and their families and friends are rarely trained observers of functional status or the many clues to functional status that can be found. Consequently, agencies rely on professional assessments even though the professionals may have had little contact with the client in their actual home context. Problems associated with professionals assessing clients in a context of illness and in curative situations (such as hospitals) are well-documented and constitute the genesis of the trend towards in-home assessments. In any case, reliable data on how clients could and would function in a given environment is hard to find. It is also expensive information to get if special assessments are needed.

For example, it is not unusual for family members to be involved as spokespersons for their elder members when some crisis arises, such as an accident or medical episode. But family members may actually know very little about the day-to-day details of the elder's life because they live some distance away and/or the elder tells them that everything is fine when it is not. Nutritional habits are notoriously difficult to gain accurate information about. The dehydrated elder with a potassium deficiency, which is in turn a result of poor nutritional habits while taking diuretics ("water pills"), may have been telling their family that they've been eating wonderfully well, that their weight loss is due to exercise and that their confusion is due to "old age." If that nutritional problem exists, family members may not know it, or if they discover it, understand why it exists. A neighbor, on the other hand, may have noticed behavioral changes that signal the onset of depression or have noticed that their friend is unusually withdrawn, or has sustained a significant loss.

Any and all of this information is crucial to weaving together a successful care plan in the community or in finding an optimal "match" in an alternative living setting. For the caseworker, the problem stems from incomplete and/or inaccurate information provided by well-meaning but untrained observers and masked or withheld by clients under emotional stress.

Informational Problems and the Clients

In addition to problems of poor information from formal and informal collateral informants, clients themselves are notoriously poor providers of accurate data on their conditions. Barriers may include language, a lack of knowledge pertinent to their circumstances, and idiosyncratic expressions owing to ethnic and other sociocultural influences, and, most frequently, communication and cognitive dysfunction resulting from medical conditions and/or treatments. Confusion of the over-medicated patient is a routine experience for any practitioner. It may be compounded by the disorientation and depression commonly encountered among older persons in institutional settings. Professionals in the institution probably have only seen the person when they are sick, and they may have strong tendencies to paint a picture to an assessor which colors care-giving possibilities in medically conservative and institutional terms. Unfortunately, these professionals may also have incentives stemming from pressures to reduce lengths of stay for older patients (e.g., courtesy of "Diagnostic Related Groupings" (DRGs), or Medicare, and other reimbursement mechanisms). These pressures may encourage assessors towards short-run solutions but also contraindicate for long-run benefits for the patient. Results on the one hand would lead to unnecessary institutionalization and/or higher costs, and, on the other, to medical risks that should not be taken regardless of costs. But in either case, an objective assessor has to be able to get good judgments in spite of these problems.

Two final points regarding information from clients and family members are in order. The first is that clients and their families are usually under a great deal of stress when a caseworker is first called in. There will usually have been some significant change in their lives, brought on by a medical episode or a change in family structure which signifies some sort of loss. It is understandable that communications and judgment may initially be clouded with emotions and confusion.

A second point is that caseworkers play a significant role in how communications will go and how clear information will be. By leading clients, families, and others to the needed data, rather than expecting them to know what is needed as well as to draw conclusions on their own, the worker can assure that he or she gets what is needed. Clients and families will then understand how the situation fits together. This is to say that a skilled assessor can facilitate the collection of data and the functioning of the client and family by giving information back to them as he or she goes about collecting it. An unwillingness or inability to provide this feedback would mark a severe shortcoming in a worker's skills and the capacity of a community care system at large.

Clients' and Providers' Fears

The next two major problems spring from clients and their environments and are actually intimately related. One is clients' fears about people coming into their homes, and the other is providers' fears when working in high crime areas or in visiting clients in locations extremely difficult to get to.

A fearful client, whether they live in a dangerous area or not, presents formidable problems to case managers and care providers. Such clients present all sorts of obstacles to care providers, from refusing to allow them entry to requiring the presence of a relative or friend each time a provider is in the home. While this may seem trivial, it creates real problems if not resolved. Demands placed on informal caregivers and professionals can become enormous, not to mention the serious logistical problems, if a client develops elaborate demands for assurances that nothing untoward will occur. Clients have been known to demand, in addition to appropriate identification, telephone calls indicating that someone is coming, the presence of a family member and/or the caseworker when direct care personnel (nurses, aides, etc.) come for the first time and every time thereafter, that a worker such as a home chore worker never leave their sight, etc. This kind of demanding behavior can very easily render home care impossible because it becomes too difficult to accommodate the client's fears. If you add to it a few of the bigotries that frequently accompany this sort of personality trait, it can get to the point where providers of care will simply refuse to be involved.

All associated with home care should be concerned about the very real danger of abuse of isolated and frail older people. Research says that elder abuse is far more widespread than commonly acknowledged, and it is not something that is usually done publicly. Home care workers and caseworkers will be in and out of client's homes consistently, and should be trained to spot signs of abuse in an elder's environment. Further, they should be extremely sensitive to the fears of someone who has experienced abuse or some sort of assault in or near their home. Their anxieties are legitimate and workers should be prepared to be understanding of any obstacles that clients may present that are attributable to their experiences. Workers may even have to guard against a tendency to make light of or diminish the validity of a client's fears, which may be in part justified. But once it goes beyond reasonable efforts and prudent controls, fear can actually choke off the flow of support that is needed.

The Environment

The flip side of this coin is the problem of getting care to people in dangerous, hostile environments. When hostility comes from abusive family members, the problem can very quickly resolve itself for better or worse by the client barring the problem family member or banning the formal providers of care. Any one of those steps may be affected by the actions of civil authorities in given local circumstances. While practices vary considerably from locality to locality, the police or other law enforcement officials may be willing to impose and enforce legal sanctions on abusive persons. Occasionally, removal of an abusive person may also remove a significant source of informal care and, particularly if the authorities become involved, the emotional cost of intervention for the client will increase. It may become so high that they will not use the authorities to protect themselves.

Still more complex are environmental problems such as high crime areas or inaccessible locations. The solutions are not always apparent. Examples abound in inner-city neighborhoods of older homeowners who become frail and refuse to leave their homes. Their once safe neighborhood deteriorates and public officials become frequent targets of assaults and/or robbery. It can even get to the point where access to whole areas is controlled by gangs, a not infrequent problem in public housing projects. Occasionally, providers may even be politely, but very firmly, refused entrance.

In such cases, the client becomes hostage to larger social forces that protective service laws and other similar measures do not meaningfully affect or change. Here, the workers, their agency, and the family may have to become negotiators and ambassadors. And, although it does not always work out, something usually can be arranged. For example, the leader of the tenant's council which represented residents of a housing project in Philadelphia was contacted and convinced that older residents would suffer seriously because a gang was stopping any nonresident from entering the project. This meant that caseworkers, homemaker aides, and home-delivered meals could not get to the nearly 40 frail older residents. A deal was struck which resulted in female gang members escorting delivery personnel in exchange for seats on the tenant council for "youth group" representatives. As often as not, a solution is expensive, however, since paid escorts, whether from the provider agency, a municipal agency, or paid neighborhood personnel, are usually the final answer.

Inaccessible locations are quite another matter, however. Some locations are simply too difficult to get to under certain circumstances, such as snow storms, rain storms, and fog. In these cases, home care needs to be viewed in different terms, with more modest goals for the level of physical disability and medical care needs that can be accommodated. Cost considerations differ too, since it can be anticipated that in the absence of very capable and highly motivated informal caregivers it will cost more to do less. If barriers are more episodic, such as snow or fog, then provisions can be made for occasional inaccessibility through use of new technologies in food and communications industries. In any case, inaccessibility carries with it serious risks for the frail elderly, whose health status can change dramatically in a short period of time. Such risks must be examined carefully and undertaken only with the full cooperation and knowledge of all those concerned.

The Problem Client

A last problem encountered and difficult to plan for is the problem client. There are a number of older people who are socially isolated from family and friends because they are unreasonable, unfairly demanding, verbally or physically abusive, and/or simply hard to get along with. These people are frequently well-known even in large human service networks because they are often so demanding that they go from agency to agency in an unsuccessful search for absolute satisfaction. While these people can drive to distraction everyone associated with them, they are in some ways easier to deal with than the more subtle problems of individual personality clashes that cannot be attributed to extreme personality types. These situations require extensive discussion of very uncomfortable issues, and they test the professionalism and commitment of formal and informal caregivers alike. Some clients are more subtly manipulative, and spend a great deal of effort convincing one person of the legitimacy of their grievance against another. Such a person may seem sweet and charming to an administrative or elected official, and it is not until the problem surfaces repeatedly that a pattern can be demonstrated. While these cases seem to be relatively few, they carry a high personal emotional cost for workers and everyone else. Workers and their supervisors need to be able to rely on one another to cope with these situations when they arise.

ROLES TO COPE WITH IT ALL

In the face of all these and other obstacles, service management workers, their supervisors, and their agency administrators have a range of skills and approaches that they can bring to bear to resolve these and many other human service problems. Rather than listing and discussing specific steps, we shall discuss several ways of viewing the roles of workers and their administrative supports as they relate to the challenges presented by arranging and managing care for homebound frail elders. These conceptualizations should prove useful in placing our work and activities in an understandable context.

Bureaucratic Guerrilla Team Role

Our first role is that of a bureaucratic guerrilla team. If a service management program operates in an environment which fosters dysfunctional systems, then the problem being faced by a service management team is one of trying to engineer ways to make the system work. You have to remember two important things. First, the best work is done when good workers have good supervisors and supportive administrative leaders—hence the team. Second, any existing system will have its own vested interests. This means that bureaucratic guerrillas will have to be prepared to combat those who want to keep things the way they are without running afoul of basic ground rules that can put them out of action. Hence the idea of the bureaucratic guerrilla. As much as systems can and should be changed, even the best system will have faults and will be designed for usual circumstances rather than exceptions. A service management unit's main job is to pursue a client's best interests as they and the client best see them within the limits of reason and resources.

Broker Role

Another way of viewing the role of a service management organization is as a broker that wheels and deals on behalf of a given client and their family. In this characterization, we can see what is the real service role of a service manager. He or she brings a client's needs and resources to the marketplace and tries to find services that can match them as well as possible. As a broker, the service manager must help clients clarify goals and objectives and may have to counsel them on how realistic their expectations may be and/or which services best meet their needs.

In systems where workers manage resources directly and are held accountable for their use, a brokerage role is expanded somewhat to include representing the interests of the system you work within. Lest anyone feel that this combination of responsibilities too seriously compromises your ability to represent a client's interests because of this dual role as a manager of resources and as an advocate, it should be pointed out that all workers have constraints on what resources they can obtain for their clients. This expanded brokerage role merely gives you a greater knowledge of the true capabilities of available resources and more leverage over their use. An increased accountability that accompanies this expansion in authority, while being time consuming, is really only making the brokerage role more complete.

Advocate Role

The role that service managers and their agencies most readily identify with is the advocate role. While this is close to the "bureaucratic guerrilla" role described above, it really has a broader scope. Frail older persons, if they are to remain in their homes, need support and care from a variety of systems of care. These range from medical/health and social service systems to income maintenance and municipal services. Service managers and their agencies must be prepared to address any and all of these systems on behalf of their clients. One slightly unusual example is snow plowing in northern cities when a homebound client lives on a small residential street and relies on home-delivered meals. These small streets, often very narrow and clogged with parked cars in older sections of eastern cities, are usually among the last to be plowed, and in some cases seem all but forgotten. Whether by convincing a usually unsympathetic streets department, or by obtaining the assistance of emergency vehicles operated by the local National Guard, the case manager needs to assure that vital services can get through. But of all the roles, this one may be the most satisfying and energizing. People that enter this field usually do so with the intention of helping people, and the sense of being effective is never stronger than when an obstacle is overcome or a barrier met and broken through. Service management is frequently very frustrating and demanding. Frustrations and sense of inability to change things become heavy burdens. Advocacy functions are important to pursue in this context and an advocacy role helps to focus workers and their supervisor's energies on the rewarding goal of improving the circumstances of their clients' lives. Such positive functions can sustain people through many encounters with difficult obstacles.

Worker As Resource Role

The last role concept views the worker as a resource. To see this concept completely, we have to examine it from the perspective of the client, the system, and the individual workers themselves.

For clients, the worker is a source of advice and counsel, an advocate, and a broker. A broker is also a gatekeeper and representative of the system. This means that the worker embodies both what the system can and cannot do for them. In this light, the worker is there to tell the system what the client needs and to get the system to do what it can be reasonably expected to do to meet those needs. Particularly where a given older person's needs are complex and extensive, the worker is the resource.

From the viewpoint of the system, the worker represents a service resource and management resource. Workers either control the flow of services directly or help clients get resources through referrals thereby controlling the use of services indirectly. When utilized properly, system managers learn that service management workers can tell them how well service agencies perform. They identify where gaps actually exist, what changes can make things better, and what is going on with other systems and organizations that affect older people. Finally, service managers themselves are consumers of the systems' resources, and represent a significant cost. Many systems are designed in such a way that the numbers and capacities of service managers act as the most important structural limit on the size of the whole system. Service managers represent an important investment for the system and they need to be viewed and managed as a valuable asset.

A Cautionary Note

Service management casework is an extremely demanding job, requiring the skills of a social worker, a public nurse, a negotiator, a counselor, a secretary, and sometimes an accountant. It often puts the worker in a position where they pursue the human service goals that they came to pursue, but the exact nature of their day-to-day activities is more administrative than anything else. They also see society's treatment of older people at its worst. They may have to constantly battle with seemingly blind bureaucratic rules and limitations, hostile families, and neighbors. In the worst of all worlds, they may face administrative leadership blind to their needs and uninterested in anything but reports.

All of the work above, it should be noted, is for a client population that almost never gets well. The nature of services to the chronically impaired is to help them maximize and maintain their potential. But this is to be done in the face of inevitable decline and in spite of roles which frequently involve tremendous physical and emotionally demanding work. One must add to this the problems of poor pay, a lack of clear career paths, and few promotion opportunities. Taken together with the generally sceptical attitude of society at large toward human service roles, we have all the ingredients for stress and burnout.

Against this daunting array of challenges, workers have their own resources to use as tools to accomplish what they need. They must evaluate their strengths and weaknesses, and seek to add the skills that they lack. But most of all, they need to husband their energies in such a way as to assure that they try as hard as is needed to accomplish what can realistically be achieved without being consumed themselves in the process.

They themselves, their skills, and their efforts, are the resources that make the whole thing work or fail. Workers manage resources and control the rate at which they are consumed. They need to consider themselves in that light.

SUMMARY

Our intention is to describe some of the problems that workers and agencies can expect to encounter in providing services to the homebound elders. We have only given an overview of the range of issues that normally occur. New service management systems are being developed all over the country. These new agencies will add many caseworkers, supervisors, and administrators to the numbers already involved in this critically important work. Their experiences will someday shed a great deal more light on the ins and outs of this complex service. Service management, when carried out properly, can allow the entire system of community-based long-term care for frail elders to develop positive changes. Someday, because of service management, unresponsive rules and bureaucratic barriers to protect the system from abuse will not be necessary. Although unlimited resources for unlimited amounts of care will never exist, a system can be made to offer quality care to chronically ill older people. Care can be provided where the elderly most frequently want it and where they will likely live longer and happier lives—in their homes.

3

The Paper Trail

Kirby G. Shoaf

Too much paperwork! Everyone involved in community-based long-term care agrees too much paperwork exists. Some projects report that their case managers spend up to 20 percent of their time just on paperwork alone. As case managers quickly point out, they came to help frail elderly persons, not to fill out forms.

Several reasons explain why so much paper abounds in community-based long-term care agencies. First, these agencies perform more than just one function, unlike a relatively straightforward information and referral agency. These multiple functions include activities such as screening for eligibility, assessing needs, and planning, ordering, and monitoring services. Second, agency staff deal with client problems ranging from housing to substance abuse to incontinence to cooking—all in one day. Third, multiple funding sources demand what amounts to separate sets of accounting books for each source.

When one adds the need for accountability to these complexities one begins to see why the "paper trail" is as long and wide as it is. Accountability alone has several dimensions, each with its own documentation needs. For example, fiscal accountability demands an audit trail of services provided. Clinical accountability requires a means by which a care plan can be judged to be equitable and in the client's best interests.

Multiple functions, problems, funding sources, and accountability generate paperwork for any complex service agency. In the case of demonstration projects, an additional demand exists: research. Demonstration projects are created to show comparative results (e.g., less cost) and collecting quality data is the name of the game. With all the varied demands for different documentation it is not clear, at times, which tail is wagging which dog. And all of this occurs in the name of helping the frail elderly.

Each demonstration project has had to deal with paperwork problems (what researchers refer to as "instrumentation"). This chapter tells how our project, the Community Care Organization of Milwaukee County, Inc. (CCO), dealt with and resolved paperwork problems. We do not pretend to say that we "definitively solved" the problem. But over the last few years we developed operational answers to satisfy the various demands for different types of information. As we go along our "paper trail" think how our solutions fit your situation. From such critical thinking comes progress.

Before embarking on the "paper trail" we will give some background information on our program.

PROGRAMMATIC BACKGROUND

Community Care Organization of Milwaukee County, Inc. was established in 1977 to implement a community-based long-term care research and demonstration project. Our project was designed to develop and operate a comprehensive coordinated system of in-home and community services for functionally disabled individuals (elderly, adult disabled, and blind). As a nonprofit corporation, CCO-Milwaukee was one of the three locally administered demonstration sites in Wisconsin. Our project was funded through the cooperation of the W. K. Kellogg Foundation, the U.S. Department of Health and Human Services, and the State of Wisconsin. A Federal waiver to the State Medicaid program made many new services available to the Medicaid-eligible client.

CCO makes available alternatives to premature or inappropriate institutionalization in a nursing home or hospital. We provide a comprehensive array of community-based health and social services. We assess client needs, develop a realistic plan of care for remaining at home, and fund and coordinate individualized packages of community services. We provide no direct services except case management and contract for all services with providers on a per client, as needed basis.

All CCO clients are unable to manage their lives independently and require help with tasks essential to daily living. Without CCO's assistance the only option for many of these individuals is nursing home admission.

The CCO model borrows heavily from the "personal care organization" concept developed by the Levinson Policy Institute of Brandeis University. The notion was that many persons could be maintained at home if certain simple services were more readily and easily available. Chronic health or disability problems of many persons meant that they would need "long-term" care for the rest of their lives. If the right services were offered, further deterioration could hopefully be prevented, they could lead a reasonably comfortable life at home, and the frequently painful and upsetting experience of admission to a nursing home could be postponed as long as possible. A home care organization would assess an individual's capability of staying at home with needed community services, obtain and coordinate the services needed, and offer continuing management and monitoring of the package of community services.

To serve persons not eligible for Medicaid, CCO secured funding from the United Way of Greater Milwaukee. Our primary target group was the near poor, those whose income or assets slightly exceed the eligibility level for Medicaid. This population could not afford costs of home care services but could quickly become Medicaid eligible if placed in a nursing home. Persons of higher income could benefit from developing and monitoring a logical service package. We constructed a sliding fee scale for amount of client contribution based on the individual's ability to pay.

SERVICE PROVISION PRINCIPLES

As the CCO plan for operations was developed, we established several significant principles or policies for service provision.

Services for Functional Disabilities

In determining our approach, we were aware that many elderly are subject to multiple disabilities which are closely interrelated. Mrs. Malone, for example, at the age of 76, lived alone in subsidized elderly housing. She struggled with an amputated right foot brought on by diabetes and complicated with osteoporosis. She suffered from depression not only associated with her disabilities but from the recent death of her husband. Our assessment tool needed to be multidimensional and emphasize functional assessment. Client need was determined by functional ability and services were matched to that need.

Separation of Assessment and Service Provision

We believed it was important to separate the assessment function from service provision. We wished to avoid a vested interest situation in which a service provider must decide if a client needs a service provided by that agency. Our structure permitted CCO service coordinators to select the most appropriate provider, type, level, and amount of service. Service coordinators could truly be advocates for clients rather than advocates for a service provider.

Services "As Needed"

CCO acts as a broker for services rather than directly providing them. We established purchase of service contracts on an "as needed" basis. We did not give any block grants or guarantee any minimum. Since this differed significantly from traditional approaches in the community, we were told no service provider would enter into a contract with us. However, the prospect of new business for agencies helped to convince them to try this new approach to contracting. Perhaps owing to the adage that services follow dollars, we had no difficulty recruiting service providers.

CCO had contracts for 15 different services with a total of 53 different service providers in Milwaukee. Contracts specified service standards and allowable unit rates with each provider. Services are ordered and purchased by unit on a fee-for-service basis as needed by individual clients. Contract services included:

- adult day care
- chore service
- counseling
- home-delivered meals
- homemaker/home health aide
- housing assistance
- medically oriented day services
- respite care
- transportation / specialized
- advocacy
- companionship
- diagnosis and evaluation
- homemaker
- hospice services
- medical equipment and supplies
- nutritional education
- skilled nursing
- transportation / taxi

CCO was able to coordinate a broad array of both health and social services. CCO had the primary responsibility for coordination of all services received by CCO clients, including those services funded by other sources. Occasionally it was necessary to make an exception and permit another agency to assume the lead-agency role. At the request of a client, we frequently dealt directly with the client's doctor. Often a doctor recommended nursing home placement because no other option appeared to be available. At times, our role was to act as an advocate for the client in communicating the desire to remain living independently and in constructing an option where one did not exist.

Service Supplementation

We recognized and valued the importance of the informal support systems and sought to maximize support systems that clients already had. As a policy, we supplemented rather than supplanted existing services. A client already participating in a subsidized congregate meal site program could not receive home-delivered meals through CCO. In the development of a service plan, we encouraged active participation of the client and families or support networks. Those most closely associated with the client's situation frequently offered the best suggestions for the most effective use of CCO resources. This sometimes resulted in the negotiation of an agreement of what would be the contribution of the client, the support system, and CCO. If, for instance, an elderly client lived with her daughter, we might agree to provide a companion for two half-days each week but not for five days each week. Based on the income and assets of the client, we might request a 25 percent copayment of services purchased.

Centralized Service Coordination/ Case Management

It was originally proposed that the CCO organization contract for case management or service coordination rather than provide these services directly. We chose to provide these services through personnel employed directly by CCO. Our primary reason for not subcontracting for service coordination was the principle of separation of assessment function from service provision. Since those agencies which would be appropriate to provide case management were also providers of service, they could not be utilized. Establishing a centralized service coordination function within the CCO agency permitted a maximum degree of control, flexibility, and manageability.

This system vested responsibility with one person, the service coordinator, to coordinate services to clients from separate agencies. A service coordinator assisted the client in gaining access to components of the entire service system by providing information about access to services unfamiliar or previously unavailable to the client. A coordinator sought to organize all services into a coordinated integrated package to maintain the client's well-being and maximize his or her independence.

Service coordinators have responsibility for:

- assessment of the client's situation and needs;
- identification of services to meet those needs;
- ordering and coordinating the delivery of services;
- evaluating the adequacy of services ordered;
- provision of follow-up service monitoring to ensure quality service delivery continues;
- liaison with all agencies and family members involved;
- identification and correction of problems within the service system that prevent the client from receiving needed services; and,
- involving the client at every step of the service planning and delivery.

Service coordinators brought a variety of skills and experience to CCO from a variety of disciplines. Some of our registered nurses had psychiatric and public health experience. CCO had both Bachelor's level and Master's level social workers with experience in counseling, geriatric services, and alcohol and drug abuse. Other coordinators had education and experience in physical rehabilitation, developmental disabilities, and vocational rehabilitation.

We believe a wide range of skills of service coordinators ensures the input of different areas of expertise into client case planning. It also allows for peer review, information sharing, and mutual support. It broadens the sphere of decisionmaking for client services.

Difficult, unusual, or problematic cases are discussed and resolved with service coordinator supervisors and in multidisciplinary team meetings. At weekly staff meetings the entire team offers perspectives from different disciplines and viewpoints to aid in client service planning, developing strategies for addressing service needs, and resolving problems. We experienced a noticeable blurring of professional discipline identification as nurses acted more like social workers and vice versa. Depending on the complexity, a service coordinator's case load could vary from 45 to 70 individuals.

Client Advisory Committee

In addition to ongoing participation in their own service planning and service delivery, clients themselves have a voice in the overall operation and management of CCO through the fifteen-member Client Advisory Committee. The committee makes recommendations to the Board of Directors and the CCO staff on the quality of care provided to clients and on overall policy directions for the Community Care Organization. The Client Advisory Committee:

- represents clients' concerns regarding CCO programs;
- provides feedback regarding CCO program effectiveness, operations, and coordination;
- recommends methods of improving services to CCO clients;
- represents concerns of elderly and disabled adults in the Milwaukee community;
- identifies and defines new problems and need areas in the community; and,
- determines whether CCO is successful in meeting its overall goals and philosophy.

THE PAPER TRAIL

First Stop on the Paper Trail: Screening

Since CCO was a research and demonstration project to serve persons who would otherwise enter nursing homes, it was critical to develop eligibility criteria. These criteria would determine program eligibility and appropriateness to ensure that services were targeted to appropriate individuals. There was a danger that, if enrollment was open-ended, the program would admit persons who were in need of community medical and social services but who were not really candidates for nursing homes. If targeting were not precise, the program could not demonstrate cost effectiveness in its use of Medicaid dollars to serve nursing home candidates at home.

It was relatively simple to establish certain criteria. Eligible clients must be residents of Milwaukee County. If clients are not Medicaid eligible, they must agree to a copayment percentage based on their income and assets. A client needed to be at least 65 years old or disabled. If disabled, the client needed to be older than 18 and certified as disabled. We accepted as certification receiving benefits from Social Security, Supplemental Security Income, or Veterans Administration programs. Two-thirds of the clients enrolled were over 65 and one-third were adults who were disabled or blind.

The issue of developing a criterion for imminence of institutionalization was a more difficult decision. Theoretically, it is possible for anyone to remain in their own home if enough home care resources are made available. An upper limit for projected direct service expense was established. Frequently, this information was not known until the full functional assessment was completed. Homemaker/home health aide services were rarely provided more than three times per week.

"Service needs too great" became a reason for ineligibility when projected direct service expense exceeded comparable nursing home expense. Exceptions were sometimes made to allow for a time-limited service plan with specific objectives. Recuperation following an acute episode or hospitalization could easily warrant daily home health aide visits on a temporary basis.

Our research design required some determination of imminence of institutionalization. We agreed that no existing instrument could accurately predict which persons would otherwise be institutionalized. To partially deal with this problem, researchers proposed establishment of a randomly selected control group. While control group establishment greatly enhanced the validity of evaluative findings, it did not assist in the determination of who should be served by CCO.

Preadmission screening for nursing homes in the Milwaukee area did not exist even on a voluntary basis. We found instruments which identified persons as having the typical nursing home profile to be unacceptable. In addition to believing that a large percentage of nursing home placements were inappropriate, we knew that many people with impairment equal to nursing home patients existed in the community.

Our research of literature identified a consistent set of factors associated with the nursing home placement decision:

- physical functioning;
- social resources and relationships;
- mental and emotional status;
- physical environment;
- financial situation;
- medical condition; and
- attitudes toward institutionalization.

While we knew these factors were associated with placement, we knew much less about the relative importance of each.

The Geriatric Functional Rating Scale (GFRS), developed by Dr. H. Grauer of McGill University, was selected as the most reliable screening instrument available for the specific purpose of nursing home eligibility (Grauer & Birnbom, 1975). The GFRS became the core of our screening process. Selection of the GFRS as the screening tool was influenced by its proven validity and predictive ability.

GFRS assesses a client's physical and mental disability, and takes into consideration functional ability and support available from community or family resources. Plus and minus point values are assigned for functioning ability of: physical condition, mental condition, support from the community, living quarters, relatives and friends, and financial situation.

Researchers who developed the scale established the following score values:

- persons with a score above 40 were capable of living in their own homes;
- a score between 20 and 40 indicated that the person required some supportive care but not necessarily in a nursing home; and,
- a score under 20 indicated that care was required in a nursing home or other intensive care facility.

Since CCO wanted to target a group most eligible for nursing homes and those most in need of home care services, most clients were required to have GFRS scores below 20. Since it was likely that some persons with scores above 20 would need nursing home placement if home care services were not available, a provision for exception was established. If someone scored above 20 they could be eligible for services if the service coordinator could adequately document a need for CCO services. Of all clients enrolled in the program, 78 percent had GFRS scores below 20.

Typically, the screening process was completed over the telephone in less than 15 minutes. In some cases, further investigation was necessary to determine if a potential client met eligibility criteria. A service coordinator would then meet with the applicant and family, usually at the potential client's home, to obtain additional information. Intake workers (paraprofessionals) performed the telephone screening process, later verified by a service coordinator.

GFRS received some initial criticism from the community because it allegedly did not provide for specific disability groups and was seemingly arbitrary in the assignment of point values. We defended the GFRS on the basis that it was the most reliable instrument available. A follow-up survey showed that not only is the GFRS applicable to a wide variety of disability groups but proved to have good predictive capabilities. In the control group, a strong correlation existed between the lower GFRS scores and the higher numbers of nursing home placements (or deaths).

At the time of CCO program start-up we visited many agencies and organizations in Milwaukee to establish a referral network by explaining CCO services. We held separate orientation sessions for hospital, community agency, and nursing home representatives. Over 400 people were informed about CCO purposes and services through these sessions. Represented were all 22 acute care hospitals, 85 community agencies, and 18 out of 64 nursing homes.

We explained we were not going to unconditionally expand human services but rather to test a coordinated and managed community-based service model. We assured nursing home administrators it was not our purpose to put nursing homes out of business. We also expressed our desire to work with nursing homes in an attempt to utilize their facilities more appropriately.

Public service announcements on television and radio, and in local newspapers brought referrals directly from clients and their families. Since the majority of nursing home admissions are through the acute care hospital, we concentrated efforts on informing the social service departments and discharge planners of all community general hospitals. Interestingly, while the most appropriate referrals were from hospitals, the greatest number of referrals came from community agencies. Given that nursing home admission often follows a hospitalization, we found referrals from hospitals usually met our program eligibility criteria. Community agency referrals were often simply seeking a possible funding source for their own services and we determined nearly one-third of these referrals to be ineligible for the CCO program.

Second Stop on the Paper Trail: Assessment Instrument

Searching for the perfect assessment tool is akin to the search for the meaning of life. We struggled with analyzing strengths and weaknesses and limitations of many different assessment instruments. We attempted to balance the required length of time to complete an instrument and the level of expertise required to obtain information needed to accurately determine service need. We questioned how we could gather subjective information and convert that information to service package needs. We struggled to weigh the importance of assessing for clinical purposes and for research and evaluation purposes.

Finally, we concluded that no perfect assessment instrument existed. We further concluded that while it is a very important part of the assessment process, it is only that, a part. It was helpful to put the assessment tool in a proper perspective. The assessment tool is a systematic method of bringing together a wide variety of information to assist the determination of need for services. Many different instruments would serve this purpose.

At one end of the spectrum was a lengthy, highly structured, forced choice questionnaire which purportedly could be administered by a paraprofessional level assessor. At the other end was a blank sheet of paper and a professional who was skilled in assessing physical, mental, and social functioning. We believed that any assessment tool or process would require our assessor to use judgment, not only in gathering subjective information but in interpreting the significance of those data. Since judgment was required in our assessment, we decided service coordinators would receive special training and we would require a professional with at least a Bachelor's degree.

In addition to searching for an assessment instrument that met our clinical requirements, we wanted to fulfill our needs for an internal management information system and the needs of an external research team. We could further posit that the instrument would be multidimensional, emphasize functional ability, and be relatively easy to administer.

The Older Americans Resources and Services (OARS) questionnaire developed by the Duke University Center for the Study of Aging and Human Development met most of our requisites (Duke University, 1978). The multidimensional functional assessment questionnaire version of the OARS instrument contains 92 questions and is designed to be administered in approximately an hour. The OARS provides information about functional ability in five areas:

- social resources: frequency and quality of social relationships with friends and family;
- economic resources: adequacy of income;
- mental health: presence of psychiatric symptoms or intellectual impairment;
- physical health: extent of physical activities and presence of physical disabilities; and,
- activities of daily living: capacity to perform various activities to permit independent living.

Responses to the questions in each area formed the basis for a functional status in each area along a six point scale. A cumulative impairment score could be obtained by adding the impairment points for each area.

During our two-year demonstration phase of the CCO program, service coordinators administered the OARS 1,143 times. In addition to gaining proficiency, service coordinators had many opinions about the instrument. Initially, coordinators complained about the length of the instrument. They seemed to be persuaded that the length was appropriate when it was pointed out that any assessment tool will take time to administer by virtue of the amount of disparate information needed to be collected for an effective client assessment. The OARS provided a systematic method of obtaining useful information and often indicated areas in need of further exploration. Coordinators found the wording of some questions awkward and sometimes confusing to the client. Training videotapes prepared by Duke University were a valuable training aid for service coordinators. We felt the OARS was weak in physical health determination and we developed supplemental questions. Coordinators also felt that the mental health scale was not accurate and that the concern given to cognitive functioning was inadequate.

We were satisfied that OARS provided useful information for our case manager, research evaluator, and program administrator.

Also, OARS provided us with a consistent method for obtaining information in a fashion that permitted comparison among clients.

Service coordinators did feel that OARS called for a good bit of subjective interpretation in constructing each impairment category. They felt the summary of each impairment category was good but that the cumulative impairment score was not as relevant because it assumed equal value for each impairment category.

After working with OARS for over two years, CCO joined with a state agency to develop a functional assessment instrument. The Wisconsin Long-Term Support Project questionnaire borrows heavily from the OARS instrument and benefits from experiences gained through the assessment process of CCO (CCO, 1981). This hybrid instrument provides information along a five-point scale for levels of functioning in eight categories:

- physical health;
- activities of daily living/physical self-maintenance;
- activities of daily living/instrumental tasks;
- emotional functioning;
- social participation;
- informal support system;
- physical environment; and,
- cognitive function.

After each of these categories, the assessor is asked whether that aspect could be substantially improved within a year with appropriate treatment or training. The assessor is also asked if that aspect could substantially worsen within one year. This instrument continues by asking questions in four additional areas:

- employment and education;
- economic resources;
- communication skills; and,
- behavioral characteristics.

Our service coordinators find this instrument markedly easier to administer. They comment that the questionnaire flows better and the wording is more easily understood, and that the instrument is more thorough and calls for a somewhat less subjective interpretation. They also believe it offers an improvement in determining emotional functioning and more appropriately separates out cognitive functioning. Ironically, no complaints were made by service coordinators about the length of this instrument even though it was slightly longer than the OARS. In part, this was because sections not pertinent to a client were designed to be skipped. Additionally, service coordinators emphasized the intact support systems and attempted to strengthen them where possible. Coordinators assessed all contributions made by the client, family, and friends that enabled the client to presently live at home. Coordinators also sought the client's perception of his or her problems and needs.

Our assessment instruments are completed by interviewing clients and, if necessary or appropriate, their family members or friends. Our assessment always includes a home visit. Additional information from other agencies was obtained if a client was currently receiving or had received services. Coordinators also determined whether CCO could adequately and reasonably meet the individual's needs. A potential client was not enrolled if he or she already received well-planned comprehensive case management services or had extremely complex or difficult circumstances beyond what was considered a safe situation. Referrals from hospitals and nursing homes were considered priority with assessments completed through a personal visit within 72 hours.

Administration time for the assessment instruments was approximately one hour. Our entire assessment process, however, could last as long as four hours, depending on clients' abilities to respond or the complexity of the assessment. Frequently, assessment instruments would identify an area which required more specialized assessment. Physical therapy, occupational therapy, speech therapy, or psychiatric consultation was ordered on an as needed basis.

Third Stop on the Paper Trail: Service Plans

Three principles formed the basis for service planning and ordering:

- access: providing information on service availability and location;
- integration: assuring effective meshing of services; and,
- accountability: guaranteeing quality and continuity of services received.

After an assessment was completed, the service coordinator developed a service plan at a meeting with the client and, as appropriate, members of the client's family or friends. A plan identified areas of care in which the client needed assistance, services to be received, and agencies that would provide them. A determination was made of how CCO services could supplement client needs unmet by the client's existing support system. Coordinators then identified best options available to address unmet needs. Staff from other agencies already involved in the provision of service were involved in the service plan development. Throughout this process, services not funded by CCO but still available to clients were included in the plans. The client was encouraged to express his or her service needs and preferences.

To assist service coordinators, we developed a service ordering protocol. This protocol listed each service and how each could be appropriately used. For example, advocacy could be used for assistance to become Title XIX, Medicaid, eligible. Individual service coordinators had the discretion to order services without prior approval within prescribed limits. For example, a coordinator could order one-time chore services up to $125 without supervisor approval. Our protocol also identified potential contraindications and duplications of service. If respite care was a major goal of the service plan, adult day care services might be limited in days or hours. Depending on the situation, home-delivered meals might not be allowed in addition to homemaker services.

Occasionally a client's condition or situation was either unclear or doubtful. When a possibility existed for continued maintenance in the home, CCO would sometimes provide services on a trial basis. We would propose a time-limited trial period in which specific goals were identified. This could take the form of a gradually decreasing amount of home health aide services. A reassessment at a given date was done to determine if services should continue. Client service plans were thoroughly explained to clients or families before services started and the client or family was asked to sign a written agreement.

Fourth Stop on the Paper Trail: Service Orders

After clients and coordinators had agreed on types and amounts of services, coordinators used information gained from our assessment process to contact relevant providers. Coordinators took into account clients' demonstrated needs for services and service availability. Clients' preferences for one agency over another, especially as a result of a client's previous experience with an agency, was acknowledged. In choosing a service provider, coordinators needed to be aware of the specialization and experience of an agency relative to the client disability. Coordinators became aware of individual agencies' abilities to respond to the complexity of particular types of service needs. For example, some agencies only served a specific geographic area.

Since purchase of service contracts was established with provider agencies on an as needed basis, services could begin almost immediately after assessment. Services were normally ordered by telephone and confirmed by a written service order. Client needs for services do change over time. Revisions of a service plan are mutually agreed upon and modifications are made in consultations with client, family, and friends. A service plan must be considered a flexible document, subject to revision whenever indicated by change in any circumstances of the client.

CCO encourages client independence in service selection and self-management. Clients are encouraged to express needs and preferences for particular services, service providers, and specific levels of service. Throughout the assessment, service planing, and service delivery processes, we consider as critically important the roles of family and neighborhood in providing support, assistance, and comfort to each individual client. Families, friends, neighbors, community organizations, religious institutions, and self-help groups are usually dependable sources of help for most clients. We are committed to identifying these support networks in the assessment of clients' situations. CCO relies on that network to continue its support and to supplement networks with professional helpers only when necessary. We work toward strengthening and reinforcing both traditional and nontraditional client community support systems. Displacement of a client's support system by professional purchased services is consciously avoided. Close relatives, friends, and neighbors form the core of the traditional support system. Its value and role are reinforced by service coordinators at periodic meetings focusing on defining areas of responsibility, identifying stresses and problems encountered, and agreeing on potential solutions to those problems.

In addition to these traditional areas of support, nontraditional areas were also reviewed. Members of the nontraditional support systems are persons who give or receive support as part of their job or other social role. Taxi drivers, volunteers, drivers for home delivered meals, and other persons coming in contact with CCO clients were trained to offer emotional support by responding sensitively to clients and to be alert for any potentially critical situations. They are requested to inform CCO of any problems or difficulties observed.

Fifth Stop on the Paper Trail: Progress Notes

A major priority of our CCO program is maintenance of quality in direct services provided to clients. Information about actual delivery, adequacy, and quality of services is provided from the following sources:

- CCO clients themselves;
- family members of CCO clients;
- service personnel working with the clients (nurses, home health aides and homemaker chore workers); and
- client's record (written assessment information and progress notes).

Given the ages and disabilities of CCO clients, individuals are often vulnerable to medical crises, overall decline in their health, subtle changes in their ability to care for themselves, and changes in their economic situation. CCO must guarantee that all services provided are responding to these often frequent fluctuations. All of this ongoing information is recorded in progress notes which form an essential part of the client's record.

Typically, a client is the first person who notices difficulty or changes, but family members are also often sensitive to sudden or gradual decline. Visiting nurses, homemakers, or companions who see clients every day or several times a week are also observant regarding slow or sudden fluctuations in physical, mental, or social health, or ability to care for one's self. Any complaints, changes, or unmet needs are called to the attention of service coordinators by the client, family member, or visiting provider and noted in the progress notes.

Service coordinators regularly contact clients at least once a month, either by telephone or by visiting in person. In addition, coordinators visit a client's home at least once every three months in order to directly reassess the client's situation. Coordinators might order more or less services or a different type of service based on any number of changes in the client's total situation. For a client who had relied on a neighbor for running errands and light housekeeping but who moved away, CCO would likely provide a homemaker for four hours every two weeks. All of this information finds its way into clients' progress notes.

Both client and provider-related information is included in progress. CCO conducts annual provider performance reviews and can respond immediately to any complaints or problems regarding a particular service person. We direct particular attention to resolve any difficulties to the mutual satisfaction of client, provider, and service coordinator; resolutions must be aimed at ensuring the best care for clients. If a provider continues to offer unsatisfactory care, CCO has the design flexibility to stop utilizing that agency or service person. Much of this information is gleaned from the progress notes. After repeated failures of an agency to provide reasonable or expected quality of service, a service coordinator could simply change agencies. Since that agency may also have many other CCO clients, it would tend to be very responsive to our concerns or complaints.

Instrumental Detours

Another assessment instrument used during the demonstration period was the Areas of Care Evaluation (ACE) which was developed by the Wisconsin Division of Health as part of the level of care evaluation for nursing home residents. The ACE provided additional documentation for activities of daily living such as eating, dressing, and bathing. The notion of the research team was that this evaluation would be the same as a part of the evaluations used for nursing home residents. As one learns by hindsight, more is not necessarily better. Questions in the ACE were essentially duplicative of those asked in the OARS.

Another detour was related to measuring quality of life. One of the stated objectives of the CCO demonstration project was to increase the quality of life of clients served by CCO. Knowing that quality of life would be difficult to measure, we naively believed that we could accomplish this measurement by focusing on the client's perception of his or her quality of life. We selected a scale that was developed by the Institute for Social Research at the University of Michigan. We tested clients at the time of entrance to the program and again every six months. We used a seven-point response scale which proved confusing if not unworkable. Not only was the administration of this tool difficult, it seemed as though clients were influenced more by whether it had snowed or whether the Social Security check was late rather than by CCO services. We concluded that it may well be impossible to accurately measure quality of life. Parenthetically, over time the quality of life for both CCO clients and control group deteriorated.

We consider these "instrumental detours" to be unfortunate consequences inherent to community-based long-term care agencies since all these agencies share the common characteristic that they are new. They are just now evolving into stable organizations. As evolving entities we find out what works and what does not work only through experience. Unfortunately, we expend a lot of energy in making mistakes as well as in defending them. We should be aware that we are involved in a new field and such detours are a concommitant adjunct to progress.

SUMMARY

Major documents that make up our paper trail are:

- screening instrument;
- assessment instrument;
- service plan;
- service orders;
- progress notes.

Looking back since we first started, not one of these documents has gone unchanged. Each one developed to fit special needs and unique situations. On the other hand, these documents reflect the major functions of any community-based long-term care agency: client selection, needs assessment, service planning and ordering, and monitoring. Any community-based long-term care agency will have to deal with the appropriate instrumentation necessary to carry out these functions. That case-carrying staff devote a significant amount of their time, up to 20 percent in some cases, to the "paper trail," is not surprising. Perhaps this is not pleasing, but paperwork "goes with the territory" of community-based long-term agencies.

REFERENCES

Community Care Organization. *The Wisconsin Long-Term Care Support Questionnaire*. Milwaukee, Wis.: Community Care Organization of Milwaukee, Inc., 1981.

Duke University Center for the Study of Aging and Human Development. *Multidimensional Functional Assessment: The OARS Methodology*. Durham, N.C.: Duke University, 1978.

Grauer, H., and Birnbom, F. A geriatric functional rating scale to determine the need for institutional care. *Journal of the American Geriatrics Society*, 1975, *20*, 472–476.

4

The Ten Commandments of Case Management During Hospitalization: A Practice Perspective

Becky Peters[1]

"The Ten Commandments of Case Management During Hospitalization" have evolved from several years of case management experience in Santa Cruz County, California, a rural county with a population of 24,900 persons 65 years old and older. Santa Cruz is fortunate to have two community-based long-term care agencies. Both agencies provide comprehensive health and social services to frail elders and both use a public health nurse and social worker team to promote maximum independent living for their clients.

The primary differences in the agencies rests in the client population served by each: the Multipurpose Senior Service Program (MSSP) is a public agency supported by Title XIX (Medicaid) and State General Funds. MSSP serves 100 Medicaid (Medi-Cal in California) eligible elders who have multiple problems and could be approved by Medi-Cal for placement in a nursing home, either in a Skilled Nursing Facility (SNF) or in an Intermediate Care Facility (ICF). The other agency, LIFESPAN: CARE MANAGEMENT FOR ELDERS, is a private agency without restrictive eligibility criteria. LIFESPAN is utilized by older adults and their families to obtain and arrange cost effective, high quality, and appropriate health and social services for elders with self-care problems.

To illustrate the "Ten Commandments" we use case studies from both MSPP and LIFESPAN. Regardless of the income level

[1] The author acknowledges the assistance and consultation of Kathy Dunn, B.S.W., in the preparation of this chapter.

of the frail elder, the "Ten Commandments" will serve to help timely hospital discharges when followed by the case management team.

1. Thou Shalt Not Stop Case Management During Hospitalization

In earlier experiences as case managers, we were fearful of entering into the hallowed hospital system where we felt powerless to affect our client's condition or fate. As the focus of community-based long-term care was the home and the client was in another form of care, we often lost contact with him or her. Many times clients were literally lost through unnecessary nursing home placement because the case management team did not intervene in the acute care setting.

For example, Mrs. Reilly is a 79-year-old widow with mild to moderate memory impairment related to a nonspecific organic mental disorder. Although she lived alone, she had a gentleman friend next door who daily put her on the bus to a senior activities center. We also had other supports in place including a daily homemaker, weekly nurse monitoring, and weekend meals on wheels. Consequently, she was functioning adequately in her own environment. However, every month during her doctor's appointment, the physician became angry because she was still living at home instead of "in a nursing home where she belongs." When Mrs. Reilly was hospitalized for a biopsy, she was immediately discharged to a nursing home. Then we could not get orders for her discharge from the physician. Thus, a woman was inappropriately placed in a nursing home because a minor hospitalization stopped the case management process for three days. Consequently, we no longer become invisible in the acute care setting, having realized that case management is long-term and must follow the client to any level of care.

2. Thou Shalt Communicate with the Hospital Discharge Planner

Establishing a relationship with the hospital discharge planner (HDP) is crucial to case management during a client's hospitalization. Since there are only three hospitals in Santa Cruz County and people know each other, we have not encountered any major problems in building a reciprocal relationship with discharge planners. The key lies in establishing an ongoing relationship instead of working in a haphazard manner creating conflict and communication problems.

During our initial meeting with each hospital, we determined what our discharge planning role would be with each hospital. One of the hospitals preferred that our agency perform the discharge planning functions, including communication with the physician, ordering equipment, arranging for home health care, etc. Another hospital chose to execute all discharge planning functions for our clients with the case manager as an advisor on the sidelines. Both arrangements are effective in allowing us to continue a problem-solving relationship with our client.

When a client enters the hospital, we immediately call the HDP to alert him or her of our involvement in the case. We communicate information about the home environment, client problems, and our goals for the client. HDP then records the information in the client's chart. In this manner, discharge planning begins early in the client's hospitalization and a case manager is involved at the start.

For example, Mrs. Thomas lives in a Senior Citizen Housing Project. She has a history of manic depressive psychosis complicated by poor compliance to her medication regimen. She was managing well with a daily homemaker to set up medications until she fell and broke her arm. Upon hospitalization, we called the HDP, alerting her to Mrs. Thomas' current status. We decided to look for a temporary live-in worker since Mrs. Thomas would not be able to function adequately with her arm in a cast. We also communicated this idea to the discharge planner to follow through and complete the link. Consequently, Mrs. Thomas was only hospitalized for two days and was discharged to her home with increased home help. Without our early and ongoing communication with the discharge planner, she would have gone to an Intermediate Care Facility.

3. Thou Shalt Provide Support for the Hospitalized Client

When our clients are hospitalized, we visit them daily. Older people are especially vulnerable in total institutions like hospitals, and reassurance from the case management team is invaluable in reducing the client's anxiety and in preventing unnecessary trauma. We also keep the client up to date on discharge plans. Often a client becomes discouraged and depressed during hospitalization. We can help to keep him or her motivated and goal-oriented.

For example, Mr. Samuels, a 91-year-old widower, was hospitalized for gastrointestinal bleeding and possible cancer. He was weak, anemic, and frightened. On the second day of his hospital stay, he refused all tests, which exasperated his physician and nurses. When we visited, he reported that no one had explained the tests to him. A technician just "appeared to take me away, and I thought I was going to surgery." Immediately, we investigated the situation. After explaining to him in detail all of the tests and the test schedule, he agreed. His diagnosis was intestinal polyps, and he was discharged in three days. Our ongoing monitoring in the hospital setting thus helped an early discharge and aided communication between the hospital staff and the patient.

4. Thou Shalt Maintain the Client's Home During Hospitalization

Miss Lance is a chronic obstructive pulmonary disease (COPD) patient who was hospitalized with a respiratory infection. After we called the hospital discharge planner to inform her of Miss Lance's admission to the hospital, we made a hospital visit. We were surprised to discover that Miss Lance was expressing resistance to being hospitalized, which was increasing her respiratory distress. We discovered that the physician was considering a move to the Intensive Care Unit. Miss Lance was worried about her dog whom she had lived with for 14 years. After we promised to feed her dog twice a day, she relaxed and began to benefit from treatment. She eventually returned home to her dog.

Clients often worry about matters at home. Sometimes they worry about a disabled spouse or siblings. Sometimes it is fear of the house being burglarized. They may have forgotten to turn on the emergency alarm system, or sometimes a pet may be the problem, as in the case of Miss Lance. As case managers we usually can clear up these unsettling problems if we stay involved during hospitalization and remain sensitive to the home setting.

5. Thou Shalt Monitor the Client's Hospital Care

When a client enters the hospital, sometimes important health or social information is not communicated or is lost in the admission shuffle. The result is that the hospitalized elder suffers unnecessarily. Hospital staff may not only lose information but may cease to think in terms of rehabilitation for a hospitalized elder because "he's just old." This lack of a rehabilitation plan may come from myths about aging. It is surprising how many times the phrase "he's just old" is heard from health professionals who are dealing with confused, incontinent, or immobile elders. As case managers, we must be present to inform hospital staff of clients' prior levels of functioning and to insure that health care is coordinated and well-informed.

For example, Mrs. Meagan has two physicians, a general practitioner and a cardiologist. Rather suddenly she was admitted to the hospital with a nonfunctioning pacemaker battery. Our case management nurse was present during the admission to inform the staff nurse regarding Mrs. Meagan's other health problems and medications. However, the information regarding Mrs. Meagan's chronic bowel problems was lost and she had a severe attack of diverticulitis because she had not received her bowel medications. The attack resulted in an extra three days of hospitalization because the case managers did not monitor hospital care.

Another common problem occurs when older hospitalized patients are not ambulated early enough. This lack of ambulation results in a patient too weak to return home. We consistently monitor the client's mobility and communicate with the staff nurse, the physician, or the hospital discharge planner if the client is not getting out of bed. This too can prevent unnecessary institutionalization.

6. Thou Shalt Recommend the Appropriate Level of Care

Hospital discharge planners and the case management staff are probably more knowledgeable about levels of care than any other health professional. When deciding on the level of care or place of discharge, there are many factors to consider. These factors include the client's support system, his or her wishes, the amount of care he or she needs, the financial situation, availability of nursing home and residential care beds, and community resources. All of the factors are weighed and measured in determining a discharge plan.

The presence of our case management team and our willingness to take responsibility for a client often enables the client to return to a lower level of care. A lower level is less expensive and less restrictive for the client. We consistently make our recommendation known to the hospital discharge planner, who can then communicate with the physician. When we meet resistance from physicians, we often negotiate by agreeing that discharge to home will be a brief trial period, and if there are significant problems, the client will be placed at a higher care level. If a physician continues to resist, we may then negotiate for a short institutional stay with the stated goal being home care or a lower level of care after one month. When in doubt, we tend to choose the lower level of care.

For example, Mrs. Franks was hospitalized with chest pain. She is an 89-year-old widow with multiple problems who had been living at home with 24-hour care. She has a history of schizophrenia and hostile, belligerent behavior. Before hospitalization, she was falling, experiencing dizzy spells, and losing weight. During hospitalization, she was diagnosed with coronary artery disease and mild angina. The physician recommended a nursing home placement but, knowing her behavior problems, we feared that she would have difficulty in a nursing home. The only alternative left for this type of patient is the locked psychiatric facility which is not a pleasant alternative. So we bargained with the physician for a one month trial at home with 24-hour care and frequent nurse monitoring, the cost of which is roughly equal to the cost of nursing home care.

Not without difficulty, Mrs. Frank passed the one month probation and continues to live at home with a good deal of home help.

7. Thou Shalt Maximize the Benefits of Hospitalization

Sometimes homebound elders do not receive necessary medical workups because of difficulties with transportation, inability to tolerate outpatient testing, and the fear of leaving home. When these clients enter the hospital for an acute illness, we can insure that all unfinished business is done. Two examples follow.

Mr. Richie is an 83-year-old retired teacher who has resided in residential care for one year after he was moved from his mobile home because of "eccentric" behavior and confusion. Usually a computerized axial tomography (CAT) scan of the brain is performed when a person's mental status changes in order to rule out treatable illnesses such as brain tumors or brain abscess. But in Mr. Richie's case, he refused a CAT scan and his condition was never fully diagnosed. When he was hospitalized one year later for pneumonia, we called the physician to remind him to order the CAT scan. This time the scan revealed a benign tumor which was subsequently removed.

Another example illustrating the strategy of maximizing the benefits of hospitalization is Miss Italo. Miss Italo has severe Alzheimer's disease and bilateral cataracts. For several months we noted that her vision was decreasing and a noticeable amount of eye strain was occurring. However, we were concerned about the effects of hospitalization on this mentally disabled woman. When she was suddenly hospitalized for abdominal pain, we notified the ophthalmologist who coordinated with the primary physician. Cataract surgery was accomplished without the need for a second hospitalization.

As described in the above two cases, hospitalization can have hidden advantages when case management continues and care is coordinated.

8. Thou Shalt Encourage Early Discharge

Early hospital discharge is cost effective and reduces chances of hospital-acquired complications such as infections and falls. As one physician so aptly states: "The longer the older person stays in the hospital, the more we find wrong." We might also add, "And the more that can go wrong." Presence of the case management team in itself encourages earlier discharge. At times, it may take several days to set up services and we try to start making arrangements as early as possible to hasten discharge. Insuring that the client is being mobilized also encourages earlier discharge by keeping the client from becoming too weak for a hospital exit.

For example, Mrs. Yates was hospitalized for recurrent diarrhea and dehydration. Prior to hospitalization she was ambulatory and slightly confused. On the tenth day of hospitalization, Mrs. Yates was still on bed rest and a discussion with the nurse revealed that she assumed Mrs. Yates to be nonambulatory before hospitalization. A telephone call to the physician mobilized this client and expedited her discharge to home.

9. Thou Shalt Begin Making Discharge Plans Early

A discharge plan starts the day of hospital admission with our first telephone call to the hospital discharge planner. Then, as the client's condition and discharge needs unfold, we begin to arrange a package of services which may include some or all of the following: live-in assistance, home-delivered meals, home health agency therapist and nurse visits, an emergency alert system, medical equipment, and increased family support.

If the physician is ambivalent towards home discharge, a presentation of our prepared package of services may tip the scale and allow the patient to go home. If services are not ready due to lack of early planning, the client may have to be institutionalized or stay in the hospital longer.

Mr. Bruno is an 80-year-old Filipino man who lives with several elderly men in a rooming house. He was admitted to the hospital with acute renal failure. It became evident that he would require ongoing dialysis three times per week. The dialysis unit is 20 miles away from his home, and he had no transportation. In addition, he had a complicated medication regimen. Compounding these problems was his overall weakness and decreased ability to perform self-care activities. Given these difficulties, the physician assumed that Mr. Bruno would go to a nursing home near the dialysis unit. However, he agreed to grant us one week to set up home services while Mr. Bruno was still hospitalized.

First we put an advertisement in the paper for a commuter who could transport Mr. Bruno in exchange for some gas money. Then we notified the In-Home Supportive Services Unit of the county welfare agency of Mr. Bruno's impending discharge. They arranged for an emergency assessment to expedite getting a homemaker. We also requested a special paramedical authorization which allows a homemaker to assist with medications if instructed by a nurse. We contacted the Visiting Nurses Association regarding the teaching needs of the homemaker and they agreed to provide that very important service. One week later we approached the physician with our plan and he agreed to discharge Mr. Bruno to home where he lived until his death two years later.

10. Thou Shalt Influence Nursing Home or Residential Care Home Placement Decisions

If our clients do require nursing home or residential care (also known as "Board and Care") placement, we make specific placement recommendations to the hospital discharge planner. As case managers we have become more and more aware of the quality of care in specific institutions, and we naturally want our clients to receive high quality care. If a client is confused, we refer to several institutions that provide especially good care for confused clients. If a client needs therapy services, some institutions are better than others. A factor we also consider is the ease with which we can work with the staff of a particular nursing or residential care home. We want to know that the staff will follow through with our suggested interventions in addition to providing quality personal care and activities. To this end, we have made an effort to visit every nursing home and residential care home in Santa Cruz County.

At times, the physician may not fully understand the criteria for placement in residential care versus nursing home care. If so, the case management team can help the physician in referring to the most appropriate level of care.

A recent example occurred when Miss Andrews, an 87-year-old woman with moderately severe senile dementia, was admitted to the hospital for dehydration and a respiratory infection. Miss Andrews had been living in residential care for two years. Urinary incontinence had been a problem for several years, and we were managing adequately with disposable incontinence aids. When Miss Andrews was hospitalized, a foley catheter was inserted due to incontinence. As she improved and was ready for discharge, the physician ordered discharge back to residential care, but residential care facilities cannot accept clients with catheters. In conversation with the physician, we recommended residential care without the catheter. He agreed.

SUMMARY

In summary, case management must continue during hospitalization to prevent unnecessary institutionalization and promote maximum independent living for the frail elder. We are sure there are other "commandments" that the reader knows from experience. Please add them to our list:

1. Thou shalt not stop case management during hospitalization.
2. Thou shalt communicate with the hospital discharge planner.
3. Thou shalt provide support for the hospitalized client.
4. Thou shalt maintain the client's home during hospitalization.
5. Thou shalt monitor the client's hospital care.
6. Thou shalt recommend the appropriate level of care.
7. Thou shalt maximize the benefits of hospitalization.
8. Thou shalt encourage early discharge.
9. Thou shalt begin making discharge plans early.
10. Thou shalt influence nursing home care or residential care home placement.

You can continue with your own "commandments."

5

Boundary Crossing: An Organizational Challenge for Community-Based Long-Term Care Service Agencies

Betty Havens[1]

WHERE DO COMMUNITY-BASED PROGRAMS FIT IN SOCIAL AND HEALTH SYSTEMS?

Community-based and addressed to the long-term care needs of clients, our programs are often viewed as atypical in the spectrum of both health and social service programs. Traditionally, the typical long-term care response from the health service sector is based on the institutionalization of "patients." On the other hand, the long-term care response from the social service sector is based on subsidizing "recipients." In this milieu, community-based long-term care programs typically respond by coordinating services based on the assessed needs of a "client" or "resident."

Community-based long-term care programs are located within, responsible to, and funded by or through the health sector in some jurisdictions, the social service sector in other jurisdictions, and both of these sectors in still other jurisdictions. This lack of uniformity is, in some cases, initiated by programs themselves and in other cases imposed on programs by traditional health and social service systems in host jurisdictions. In either case, the result adds to confusion and highlights a view that these programs are unique within a single jurisdiction and across jurisdictions.

Consequently, community-based long-term care programs do not "fit" neatly in either health or social service systems, nor do

[1] The author acknowledges with appreciation the assistance of E. Thompson, L. Fineman, and P. Olson in commenting on earlier versions of this chapter.

they "fit" well in an overarching health and social service system. Because of variability across programs, elements that are central to one program may be peripheral to another. Furthermore, program elements which must be negotiated across a program boundary with other health or social service programs by one community-based program are integral to another program and totally outside the parameters of a third program.

MANITOBA'S CONTINUING CARE PROGRAM

Our Manitoba program, which is province-wide, universal, and free for consumers, was initiated by the provincial government in 1974 and gradually expanded throughout the province by 1975. This program assesses persons requiring care whether for placement in nursing homes or for home care. We deliver services to those who remain at home. Our program is a coordinated service program which provides a broad range of services to meet the needs of persons who require assistance or support to remain at home or whose functioning without home care is likely to deteriorate making it impossible for the person to stay at home in the community. Upon identification of needs, services are organized to avoid deterioration and to maintain and enhance health. This is accomplished within established policy guidelines and through an existing departmental health and social service/health center network and in conjunction with relevant private voluntary agencies.

Our program is delivered through regional offices and suboffices and through health centers and private agencies identified within the program service delivery framework and coordinating agencies. These coordinating agencies are responsible for participating with the central program office in coordinated program planning and development and for providing coordinated quality service delivery within program guidelines.

Service delivery frameworks are based upon professionally coordinated and conducted assessments of need, care planning, and supervision of service delivery. Ongoing services provided in the home are delivered both by professionally and paraprofessionally skilled persons.

For those of any age who are referred from any source, determination of need for services is based upon a clinical, a health functioning, and a social functioning assessment. Assessment is focused to identify those who, without services, would be at risk of being able to remain at home but who, with home-delivered services, could have their care needs managed appropriately.

This program model calls for each referred person to be served primarily by one staff person called the case coordinator and for assessment and care planning to be multidisciplinary.

Program guidelines call for each person to be fully assessed including identification of those activities which the person can perform, those which family members, friends, or neighbors can realistically perform, and those which require placement of services. A care plan is developed to provide for needed services which exist within the program. When needed services are not available within the program, every effort is made to secure such services from other community sources, as part of the care plan. Services provided by the program are to be the minimum required to meet need and to foster independence. Delivery is to be organized so that services are provided by the person with the minimum skill required to perform the task.

Throughout the province, the program utilizes professional and nonprofessional skills including those of nurses, social workers, licensed practical nurses, aides, orderlies, therapists, home attendants, home helpers and personal care homemakers, volunteers, and the staff of voluntary agencies as well as civil servants and hourly paid casual employees.

SYSTEMS' BOUNDARIES AND COMMUNITY-BASED LONG-CARE PROGRAMS

Rigidity of organizational boundaries, both those of community-based programs as well as those of other relevant programs, to a large extent, determines the amount of time and energy expended by staff in crossing or negotiating for others (e.g., clients) to cross boundaries. If boundaries are rigid, energy expended is very substantial and the process frustrating to both staff and clients. If some degree of openness exists, energy spent may still be substantial, but the process is more likely challenging than frustrating.

Many examples of boundary-crossing endeavors are referred to within this chapter; however, two examples, below, will serve to set the stage for further discussion.

Mrs. Smither's Granddaughter's Wedding

Mrs. Smither, age 80, lives alone in an old apartment in the central area of the city. She has been a client of the home care program for two years. Due to severe arthritis and emphysema she is unable to do her own shopping or maintain her apartment. A therapist visits her once every three weeks to monitor her exercise program and reassess her ability to perform activities of daily living (ADL). The home care case coordinator, a nurse, considers her situation to be stable and reassesses her functioning every three months by visiting her home and receives reports from all direct service providers in the interim. The case coordinator has assigned a homemaker to Mrs. Smither for three hours twice a week to assist with meal preparation, to maintain the apartment, and to protect the health and safety of Mrs. Smither. Mrs. Smither's daughter, who lives in a neighboring suburb, does all the shopping and laundry, any heavy cleaning, and assists with meal preparation four days a week. She usually arranges to have her husband and one of her sons assist Mrs. Smither into the family car to join them for Sunday meals.

Mrs. Smither's oldest granddaughter was to be married in another city and her daughter and family wished to spend two weeks with the granddaughter—potentially leaving Mrs. Smither without anyone to shop, do laundry, or assist with the other than four meals a week prepared by the homemaker. Mrs. Smither's daughter contacted the case coordinator with a request for holiday relief while the family attended her daughter's wedding. The case coordinator wished to cooperate with Mrs. Smither's family as they were providing the vast majority of services. However, shopping and laundry are not services normally provided by the home care program. The case coordinator began negotiating with a voluntary agency that provides shopping services, a neighboring nursing home to do the laundry for two weeks, and another volunteer to pick up and deliver the laundry.

In the meantime, while waiting for a response from these agencies, the case coordinator arranged additional assistance from the homemaker. This additional assistance was one hour to assist in preparing laundry, including changing linen, and two hours on two other days for meal preparation. The Saturday meal would be prepared by the homemaker on Friday and reheated by Mrs. Smither the next day. The coordinator was able to assist Mrs. Smither's daughter in arranging for a neighbor to check with Mrs.

Smither on Saturday. The neighbors further volunteered to provide Mrs. Smither's dinner on Sunday. The nursing home responded first. The administrator agreed to have the laundry done if it could be delivered before 9:30 a.m. on Tuesday morning. This schedule was acceptable to the volunteer driver.

After a week without a response from the voluntary agency regarding shopping assistance, the case coordinator contacted the volunteer shopping coordinator again. She was told that the agency did not have additional volunteer hours available in Mrs. Smither's neighborhood and had not been successful in locating additional volunteers. The case coordinator determined that one of the agency's volunteers was a friendly visitor to a tenant in the building in which Mrs. Smither lived. The case coordinator, with Mrs. Smither's agreement, arranged to have the tenant brought to Mrs. Smither's apartment as a friendly visitor on one Friday while the volunteer friendly visitor did Mrs. Smither's shopping. When this plan was shared with the volunteer agency coordinator, the initial response was negative because the same volunteers did not normally act as shoppers and visitors. However, he agreed to discuss this plan with the coordinator of friendly visitors and their supervisor. Eventually it was agreed that a change in visiting for one week could be beneficial to the agency's client and the friendly visitor agreed to the shopping assignment for this one occasion. The agency supervisor contacted Mrs. Smither's case coordinator and a final negotiation was completed. The case coordinator was able to inform Mrs. Smither and her daughter at the end of three weeks that a holiday relief plan had been developed and she wished the daughter a happy holiday.

This example, illustrated in Figure 5.1, shows that in this case 16 individuals were involved in the rather mundane task of providing two weeks of holiday relief. To help Mrs. Smither, the case coordinator crossed and recrossed family boundaries, informal support boundaries (e.g., the neighbors) and formal support boundaries (e.g., the volunteer agency) to achieve the modest goal of assisting a family to care for its grandmother.

Mr. Sawchuk's Water, Plumbing, and Heating

Mr. Sawchuk, age 88, lives alone on a small farm at the edge of a small village. He has lived on this farm all his life, has never married, and his siblings are deceased. His only relatives, nieces and nephews, live many miles away and seldom visit except on occa-

Figure 5.1. Boundary crossing for Mrs. Smither's granddaughter's wedding.

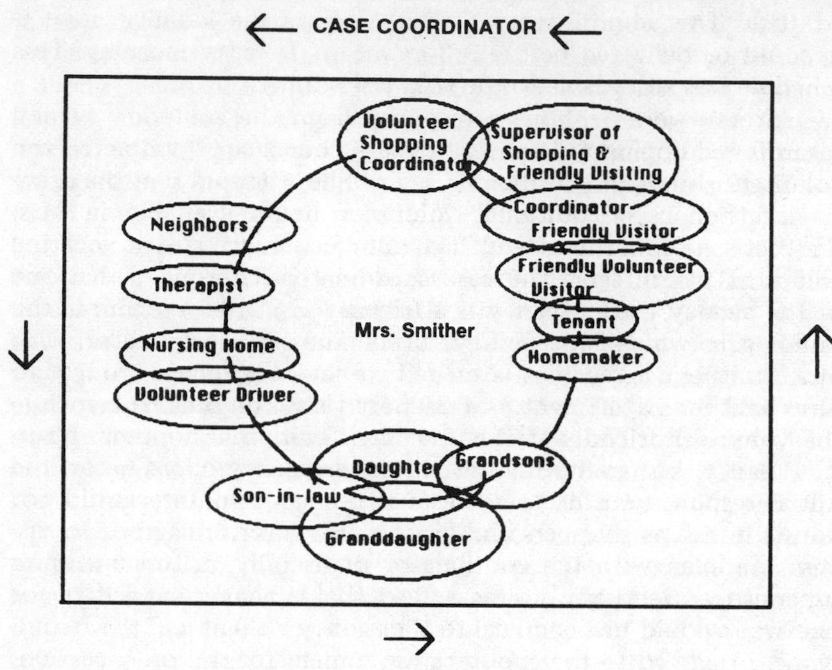

sion during the summer. Mr. Sawchuk had been coping relatively well on his farm until he suffered pneumonia last spring. Since that time, he had not been able to haul water from the well and chop firewood for cooking. He also had not built up his stock of wood used for heating in the winter. The grocer had taken to delivering supplies as Mr. Sawchuk was finding it increasingly difficult to drive to town (about 12 miles away) to do his banking and shopping.

A niece referred him for placement in a nursing home. The assessment for care indicated that he did need care but none of the staff in the neighboring nursing home spoke Ukrainian and Mr. Sawchuk spoke very little English. In any case, he did not want to leave his farm. The assessment team had grave concerns about providing home care to him without water or reliable heat in the house. Mr. Sawchuk was not opposed to having water and plumbing in the house, he had just not needed them. He had electricity for years but had not used it for heat although he had begun doing much of his cooking on a hot plate and an electric fry pan after his pneumonia-related hospital stay.

The case coordinator, a Ukrainian-speaking social worker assigned to Mr. Sawchuk, began to negotiate with the local municipality for assistance in bringing water into the house under a special senior citizen's assistance program. This took several months and many phone calls, visits, and application forms.

In the meantime, the case coordinator found a neighboring teenager who agreed to haul water from the well on a daily basis. The case coordinator also helped Mr. Sawchuk arrange with the electrical utility company to install electric heating and a hot water tank in the house with provision for the cost of the installation to be added to Mr. Sawchuk's monthly electrical bill. The grocer agreed to continue delivering his supplies on a regular basis and the public health nurse added Mr. Sawchuk to her caseload to monitor his continued recovery and general health status.

Finally, late in the fall, water was brought into the house and Mr. Sawchuk, with the help of the case coordinator, contracted with a local plumber to install a kitchen sink ordered from the Sears catalogue and attach the hot water tank. A toilet with an external septic holding tank was installed in a hallway between the kitchen and the bedroom which also served as Mr. Sawchuk's closet. Had Mr. Sawchuk required financial assistance for this latter contract, it would have meant more time and frustration in negotiating with another government agency to accomplish the task. Fortunately, Mr. Sawchuk had sold some property and farm equipment just before his stay in hospital and was able to pay the plumber and supplier.

His neighbor continues to visit Mr. Sawchuk a couple of times a week, helping a bit around the place even though the water no longer needs to be hauled. After all the work was completed, the case coordinator closed this case, as Mr. Sawchuk is able to continue living at home on his own without home care services and is no longer a candidate for an unwanted placement in a nursing home. Mr. Sawchuk and his relatives know they can contact the case coordinator if the situation changes. They say that this has given them a greater sense of security.

In this example, the case coordinator had to cross ten boundaries while he acted as a surrogate for a caring family member. This is in contrast to the example of Mrs. Smither, in which the case coordinator complemented the family's efforts.

These examples serve to illustrate the variability in degree of openness of boundaries. They also stress the importance of negotiating across multiple boundaries. No program is likely to provide all services to all clients in all situations itself.

ASSESSMENT AS A VEHICLE FOR COORDINATION AND SYSTEM CHANGE

Seldom does a client need a single service to remain in their own home in the community, so coordination of services becomes a major concern of both a providing agency and the client. If the community-based long-term care program does not include service coordination in its functions, clients or their families are left with the time- and energy-consuming task of trying to coordinate a variety of service deliverers. All of these providers are employed by and responsible to a variety of organizations. For the community-based program to coordinate health and social services from a variety of public, private, and voluntary agencies with those tasks performed by the client and his/her family, friends, and neighbors, a comprehensive multidimensional assessment is essential.

Common Assessment across Social and Health Systems

Health and social service systems vary across jurisdictions. However, given the nature of community-based long-term care programs, it is likely that components of both of these systems will be integral to any specific program and other components will remain external to these programs. Establishment of an assessment process which can be used within the program itself and with components of both systems is an essential ingredient for success.

Cases cited earlier provide examples of the importance of common assessments. Mrs. Smither's situation was shared through her assessment form and care plan by the case coordinator with the administrator of the nursing home and the volunteer coordinator of the social service agency. Neither of the two agencies had to perform a new assessment at the time of their potential involvement with Mrs. Smither. A common assessment for care at home or in a nursing home in Mr. Sawchuk's case allowed the case coordinator to determine that placement in a nursing home was neither the most suitable solution nor necessary if Mr. Sawchuk's home could be modernized. Much more effort, time, and professional staff involvement would have been required in these cases had a common assessment procedure not been in operation within the program and across system boundaries.

Assessment Based on Client and Informal Network Strengths

Assessments for long-term care normally concentrate on client weaknesses and functional deficits. However, by operating in the community from a premise of maintaining independence, assessments are more appropriately focused on strengths of the client and his/her informal support network. A portion of an assessment interview with Mrs. Beaulieu demonstrates this focus on strengths.

Mrs. Beaulieu's Assessment Interview. Mrs. Beaulieu has been referred for an assessment for care by the local public health nurse who has been visiting the Beaulieu household as part of her caseload for many years. Mrs. Beaulieu has lived with her son and daughter-in-law since she became a widow 30 years ago. The younger Beaulieus have worked all their adult lives and Mrs. Beaulieu looked after their five children as they grew up. The youngest grandchild had finished college and is about to move to another city. One of the grandchildren is married and living two blocks away with his wife and two small preschoolers. The granddaughter-in-law works three half-days a week and leaves the great-grandchildren with Mrs. Beaulieu while she works. She has noticed that Mrs. Beaulieu no longer picks up the children when they are fussing in the bed or playing on the floor. Mrs. Beaulieu has commented that she is not as limber as she used to be and has fallen several times just doing her usual tidying around the house.

During the assessment interview the nurse and social worker determined that Mrs. Beaulieu is mentally alert. She is able to get about the house, prepare meals, and generally tidy up her room, the kitchen, and help with other cleaning. Her daughter-in-law does the rest of the cleaning and the laundry and most of the ironing though Mrs. Beaulieu still irons all the linens and her own dresses. Her son and daughter-in-law do all shopping for her now, as she no longer trusts herself to walk the few blocks to and from the store alone, even to buy milk or bread. Occasionally the granddaughter-in-law brings bread or milk when she picks up her two children after work.

The assessment team was impressed with the strengths of Mrs. Beaulieu at 86 years of age and the mutual supportiveness of her family. However, they were also concerned about her reference to falls and her hesitation to walk out of doors or to pick up her great-grandchildren. They know that the family can respond to all Mrs. Beaulieu's identified needs; however, they recommended that Mrs. Beaulieu attend the nearby day hospital program for a full geriatric clinical assessment to be undertaken to determine the cause of her falls. Mrs. Beaulieu and her family felt, at that time, that she should continue her babysitting with her great-grandchildren. Following a consultation from the assessment nurse, Mrs. Beaulieu's physician agreed to make a referral to the geriatrician at the day hospital for the days when she does not babysit with her great-grandchildren. Pending the outcome of that geriatric clinic assessment, the home care assessment team made no further care plans. They forwarded their assessment findings to the day hospital, as part of boundary crossing with the medical and hospital sectors of the health system.

Assessment Identifying Weaknesses and Gaps in Support

Each of the preceding examples highlights strengths of clients and informal support networks. However, each example also identifies some weakness with the client or the informal network, either temporarily or relatively permanently. The ability of an assessment to identify the strengths initially, and then to proceed to identifying weaknesses which inhibit independence, allows the assessment team to develop a care plan and assign a case coordinator which will provide only those services which fill gaps in supporting a client's independence.

While it is essential to maintain independent functioning of the client and the support network, clearly, without these essential gap-filling services which respond to and compensate for weaknesses in a given situation, the whole situation can fall apart. When cases fall apart, no matter how small or simple the missing service is, the typical response is to seek placement in a nursing home. In most instances, the client and his or her support network can cope with an occasional gap in services or slowness in placing or replacing in-home services. But, repeated occurrences generally discourage the client, frustrate their support network, put undue burden on other formal caregivers/service deliverers and case coordinators, and may ultimately become an incentive to premature nursing home placement.

Final Assessment Process Decision: Site of Care

When a common assessment process is used across all sectors of long-term care and when the assessment itself is designed to establish types and amounts of care required, the last step in the process is to determine the most appropriate location for that care. That is, only after all strengths and weaknesses of the client and the informal support networks have been adequately assessed does the assessor begin to consider the site of care.

The importance of this order of events is most clearly demonstrated in the case of Mr. Sawchuk, who was referred to the assessment team by a niece who believed that he should be placed in a nursing home. If the team had assessed his situation on the basis of eligibility for placement in a nursing home rather than on the basis of his strengths, care needs, and his desire to remain at home, he most certainly would have been placed in a neighboring nursing home. At this neighboring nursing home no one spoke his language. A poor second choice was a nursing home many miles away where the staff and many residents spoke Ukrainian. However, the assessment revealed that, while Mr. Sawchuk required assistance and while his own home left much to be desired as a location within which to deliver services, it was possible to modify his home sufficiently to enable him to care for himself.

In addition to the "total" solution of nursing home placement and the "minimum" solution of care in one's own home there are many other potential sites of care which should be considered as options in making a final assessment decision. These include having family member(s) move into the home of the potential long-term care client, or enabling the potential client to move into the home of a family member. In some cases home sharing by unrelated individuals may also provide similar options to those involving family members. This solution is still chosen relatively infrequently among potential clients. However, as families become even more mobile and as more older adults know others who have successfully shared homes with nonfamily adults, this option may become more popular.

In some communities, it is possible to find a family which is willing to provide an adult foster home. These placements are more common than home sharing and have been especially successful and appropriate with mentally retarded and postmentally ill older adults. In many cases a family will foster two or even three older adults. Group homes may be an option in some jurisdictions. These placements generally include physically disabled older adults who have been disabled for many years. A typical group home provides a living arrangement for five to eight adults with a live-in caregiver or couple.

Senior citizens housing projects provide another potential site for providing support services. Any person living in a senior citizen's apartment may be receiving in-home services individually just like anyone else in the community. However, the presence of several persons requiring care in a single seniors complex may lead to aggregating services in ways that are not possible with the same number of people scattered in their own homes in the community. Seniors' housing projects may provide another option in making a decision about the site of long-term care.

New options are being developed all the time such as care cooperatives, board and care homes, and domiciliaries. Consequently, long-term care assessment staff and case coordinators must keep up to date on new developments and options in their own communities, to provide the broadest possible range of options to each potential client at the final stage of determining site of care.

CROSSING BOUNDARIES LEADING TO INDEPENDENCE

Maintaining the balance between supporting independence without incurring dependence is critical and seldom easy to accomplish. In an earlier example, if the case coordinator had not been committed to maintaining and supporting independence, Mr. Sawchuk would likely have been placed in a nursing home at the request of his niece. The creativeness of the case coordinator in assisting Mr. Sawchuk in modernizing his house not only allowed him to remain at home, but in fact even made it unnecessary for home care services to be provided in his home. This solution has enabled him to maintain his home, his health, and his independence.

Similarly in the case of Mrs. Smither, providing holiday relief for her daughter required the case coordinator to develop innovative strategies. Not only was it necessary to cross the boundaries of a voluntary agency with a request for shopping services, but to enable the agency to respond to the request, it was necessary for Mrs. Smither to become a substitute friendly visitor while the usual friendly visitor became a volunteer shopper for the single occasion required to keep this case intact.

The referral of Mrs. Beaulieu to the geriatric day hospital program for a geriatric clinical assessment provides another example of innovative system boundary crossing. The home care nurse assessor consulted with Mrs. Beaulieu's family physician to arrange the referral to the geriatrician at the day hospital. The clinical assessment findings will be provided to the family physician and to the home care team should follow-up services be required. In the meantime, Mrs. Beaulieu will remain at home and will continue to babysit for her great-grandchildren while she is being assessed at the day hospital. Consequently, she will be retaining her independence and continuing to contribute to her family's well-being.

In each of these examples the actual services provided may seem small, and even inconsequential. However, each service made the difference between independence and dependence. Each situation required the case coordinator to find innovative solutions to deliver services and each involved crossing system boundaries. In Mr. Sawchuk's case even jurisdictional boundaries had to be crossed. It should be noted that while the time and energy expended by the case coordinators may have seemed excessive, two factors must be considered in this context. First, these cases remained intact and the clients and their support networks were able to remain independent. Second, neither clients nor families were required to expend already limited energies in trying to coordinate services or create innovative solutions across the multiple boundaries involved. Furthermore, if it is difficult for those who know the system to make it work, it can be virtually impossible for those who do not know the system to function within it, let alone successfully cross boundaries.

BOUNDARY CROSSING LEADING TO SYSTEM CHANGES

When boundaries are crossed successfully, as defined by those on both sides of the boundary, the sectors, programs, systems, or jurisdictions become more open to further boundary-crossing efforts. The innovative solution of using Mrs. Smither as a substitute visitor and asking a friendly visitor to act as a volunteer shopper was viewed as successful by the case coordinator, by Mrs. Smither and her family, by the voluntary agency, by their client, and by the friendly visitor. As a result, both the case coordinator and the voluntary agency staff have become more open to finding innovative solutions to providing services to other clients.

Mr. Sawchuk was the first resident for whom the specific municipality had been requested to use their municipal assistance program to provide public water services to a senior. In the three years since Mr. Sawchuk's water was put in, the municipality has responded to seven similar requests and in the most recent case, water was connected just six days after the original request was filed.

When the day hospital to which Mrs. Beaulieu was referred first started doing geriatric clinical assessments, all of the initial clients were patients of the acute hospital who were about to be discharged and only three physicians were availing themselves and their patients of the assessment service. Today, the majority of the day hospital patients have never been in-patients and over 30 physicians are actively referring patients for geriatric clinical assessments.

BOUNDARY-CROSSING VENTURES

As has been suggested throughout the preceding sections, crossing boundaries is part of the stock-in-trade of community-based long-term care programs. Without a willingness to venture into boundary crossing, programs will become restrictive and boundaries will become rigid and impermeable, precluding innovative individual solutions. However, negotiating boundary crossing is not easy and tends to be both time- and energy-consuming. This section deals specifically with these ventures.

The Challenge of Making It Work

There is a certain satisfaction for a professional in successfully resolving a problem with an individual client and his/her support network. This is true when a solution is relatively straightforward and all components of the solution are readily available and internal to the program. However, it is even more challenging and satisfying when the components of the solution are external to the program. One of the components which can help many families continue to maintain care with minimal formal service supports is respite care. Respite care allows the primary caregiver(s) to do things that they must do such as banking or shopping, and other things that they wish to do such as attending club meetings, joining friends for lunch, or taking a necessary vacation. Respite care may be provided in the client's home, in a nearby nursing home, or in a hospital.

Respite Care for Mrs. Schwartz. Mrs. Schwartz is a home care client who is severely disabled with arthritis and mildly disoriented. She lives with her husband and their 62-year-old widowed daughter, who works at a nearby computer center.

The case coordinator has reviewed Mrs. Schwartz's care plan on a quarterly basis for the past four years, during which time episodes of disorientation have become more frequent. An occupational therapist monitors Mrs. Schwartz's progress in maintaining her physical functioning and a homemaker assists with household maintenance three hours a week.

As Mrs. Schwartz has become more disoriented, Mr. Schwartz has had to stay with his wife unless their daughter or the homemaker is at home. As a result, Mr. Schwartz and his daughter have found it increasingly difficult to do the household shopping, their own shopping, the shopping for Mrs. Schwartz, the laundry, and yardwork. Mr. Schwartz has also had difficulty getting to the bank. Both Mr. Schwartz and his daughter have ceased to attend social activities and seldom have contacts with friends except when they drop in to see Mrs. Schwartz or, in the daughter's case, at work. Mr. Schwartz has become less agile physically, less outgoing, and more apathetic.

As a result of these changes in Mr. Schwartz, the daughter contacted the case coordinator with a request for more homemaking time. She felt that her father was becoming less able to cope with preparing meals for her mother. The case coordinator reviewed the case and, in discussion with Mr. and Mrs. Schwartz, decided that respite care for Mrs. Schwartz would vastly improve the situation. A revised care plan maintained the three hours of homemaking and provided four hours a week of home attendant care for Mrs. Schwartz. This allowed Mr. Schwartz to do more outside the home. In addition, arrangements were made for Mrs. Schwartz to spend one week out of every six weeks in a nearby nursing home. This provided respite for both Mr. Schwartz and his daughter which enabled them to maintain more of their social contacts and to do the major tasks in their home and yard.

This solution enabled the Schwartz family to continue to care for Mrs. Schwartz for 46 weeks out of the year, with only seven hours a week of formal services. All components of this solution are within the services of the home care program, but the use of a nursing home for respite care had to be negotiated with the facility administrator and approved by the provincial funding authorities. This challenge at the boundaries of the program was successful in meeting Mr. and Mrs. Schwartz's needs. Without going outside the program, the case coordinator probably would have eventually had to oversee the permanent placement of Mrs. Schwartz in a nursing home.

The Frustration of Missing Services

In another community, in a case very similar to that of Mrs. Schwartz, a solution was more difficult because fewer resources existed. Also, while the family is larger in this next case, none of the family members live in the same community, let alone in the same household. The following description is very abbreviated, but the solution took 18 months to implement.

Finding an Adult Day Care Program for Mrs. White. Mr. and Mrs. White live in a small town and Mrs. White has been a home care client for several years due to her emphysema. More recently, she has been experiencing periods of disorientation. The nurse assigned to Mrs. White monitors her emphysema, assists with her bathing, and does her foot care. A homemaker assists with household maintenance and also meal preparation three days a week. A small voluntary "meals on wheels" program delivers meals another three days a week. The Whites' grandson and wife, who live on a farm near town, pick them up for Sunday dinner. In bad weather they bring along dinner and the great-grandchildren and spend time at the Whites'.

Mrs. White's disorientation has caused Mr. White to stay at home, as he is fearful that Mrs. White will wander off and get lost. In the winter he also worries that she may suffer frostbite. A neighbor contacted Mrs. White's nurse because he had not seen Mr. White in town for several weeks and his phone calls had been unanswered. On her next visit the nurse asked Mr. White if he had been in town recently. He replied, "I've been afraid to leave

Sarah (Mrs. White) alone since she wandered off two months ago while I was raking leaves at the back of the house." The nurse reported this to the case coordinator who visited the Whites to reassess the situation.

It became obvious that Mr. White was not sleeping or eating well and was very anxious about his wife. The grandson was doing all the shopping. Mr. White complained that no one had called and, other than an old friend who often stopped on his way to town, he had not talked to anyone in about six weeks. The case coordinator checked the telephone and discovered that the bell had been turned down accidentally. Further discussion indicated that Mr. White's hearing aid batteries were being "saved" for visits from the friend and grandson because he did not know when he would get to the city to get more.

The case coordinator, in discussion with Mr. White, decided that an adult day care program for Mrs. White at least twice a week would make it possible for Mr. White to continue caring for his wife. The problem was that the nearest adult day care program was in a neighboring town fifteen miles away. Mr. White agreed to try driving Mrs. White to the program. He did so for three weeks, at which time the roads became too icy for Mr. White to continue. The case coordinator contacted the grandson to see if he could drive his grandmother during the winter. He agreed to try. He drove his pickup truck to his grandparents' home and then took the grandparents' car to drive his grandmother to the adult day care program. This meant he drove 80 miles twice a week. After two weeks he said he simply could not continue with his farming chores, taking his children to hockey practice, and community activities, while also being responsible for driving his grandmother.

The case coordinator began negotiating with a nursing home in the Whites' home town to provide an adult day care program for Mrs. White and three other home care clients in or near the town. This negotiation took several months as the nursing home had virtually no activity programming for the residents and were very insecure about starting any new programs. The case coordinator involved the central home care program staff and the adult day care coordinator in her discussions with the nursing home staff and board.

In the meantime, a temporary solution was initiated by increasing the homemaking time assigned to Mrs. White. The homemaker prepared meals for Mr. and Mrs. White six days a week and in total spent 15 hours a week at the Whites'. This enabled Mr. White to get out more but was still not a good solution. As the weather improved in the spring, Mr. White again drove his wife to the adult day care program in the next town, at which time the homemaker was cut back to nine hours a week.

As the weather became worse again in the fall and the local nursing home had still not agreed to start an adult day care program, the case coordinator again increased the homemaker's time to 15 hours per week. By early March, the local nursing home finally started an adult day care program and Mrs. White began attending regularly three days a week. Her emphysema was monitored within the program so the nurse visited only once a month and the homemaker was cut to six hours a week. Mr. White began to take a renewed interest in the community and became a volunteer driver for the local adult day care program. He drove two other participants to the nursing home along with his wife.

Our case coordinator reports that she spent approximately 20 hours a month, for the 18 months in question, negotiating with the neighboring nursing home to take Mrs. White and another client in their program on a seasonal basis; negotiating with the local nursing home to start an adult day care program; consulting with central program staff on how to assist the local administrator in starting a program; adjusting schedules; and consulting with Mr. White and the other three spouses of clients in the same community to hold all these cases together in the absence of a service which had to be started across a program boundary. Direct service time consumed by these four clients during that 18-month period averaged 80 hours a week. After the adult day care program was in place, it averaged only 21 hours a week by using a much more satisfactory and viable solution to their situations. If the adult day care program had been available in the local facility, this would have been an easy situation to deal with rather than one which consumed much time and incurred great frustration.

The Agony of "Holding It Together" or "Watching It Fall Apart"

These last two examples, Mrs. Schwartz and Mrs. White, and to a lesser extent, Mrs. Smither, highlight the importance of the case coordinator being able to keep on top of his/her caseload. The difference between "holding these cases together" and having them "fall apart" is being able to respond quickly to changing needs and situations. Having flexible hours of service in a community-based long-term care program can make the difference in what responses are possible. In other words, being able to adjust the hours of service to a client (or clients) depends to a large extent on the case coordinator's ability to redesign care plans quickly and on her/his ability to hire staff on an hourly basis. Staff hours will therefore vary depending on the mix of cases in a community at any given time. This variation and flexibility also requires negotiating across boundaries in terms of personnel officers, unions, labor law review boards, and payroll staff.

BENEFITS OF BOUNDARY CROSSING

A client stands to gain most when the program staff, especially the case coordinators, are not only willing to cross program and system boundaries but are also successful in doing so. It is important to the client for the program to keep its boundaries as open as possible to enable boundary crossing to occur with relative ease.

It is also advantageous for the program to be adept at crossing these boundaries. In many ways, the success of any community-based program is the sum of its successful client solutions. Successful solutions are facilitated by the openness of boundaries and hence the program is more successful. It should also be noted explicitly, at this point, that success breeds further success. Each successful solution sets the stage for future successes.

Furthermore, initiatives taken to meet emerging needs, and which involve the crossing of boundaries, may lead to mutual recognition of these needs on both sides of the boundary and ultimately to new formal resource development. Examples of this evolution are found in the Manitoba development of adult day care programs and respite care programs in nursing homes. Formal programs began in 1979 and 1980, respectively, with entry through our Continuing Care Program. These two new programs had their beginnings in ad hoc arrangements similar to those initiated for Mrs. White and Mrs. Schwartz.

The broader community and relevant health and social service systems also benefit because they are more able to draw on resources and expertise of the long-term care program when boundaries are kept relatively open and can be relatively readily crossed.

As long as the long-term care program negotiates to cross others' boundaries, it also simultaneously becomes a resource to the other programs and systems and shares its expertise in the process. A functional reciprocity is established. An effective community-based long-term care program can enable other facets of these broader systems to function more appropriately and effectively. They will not be expected nor required to respond to inappropriate cases and situations once their internal capabilities are known by others.

CONCLUSIONS

The key to currently successful community-based long-term care programs, regardless of jurisdictional location and system descriptions, is successful boundary crossing based on common assessments, openness of boundaries, and willingness of program staff to create innovative individual case solutions. It is taken as fact that these programs are "mavericks" within health and social systems. It must also be expected that program staff will be committed to unique solutions and flexibility in use of direct service and other resources. Furthermore, it is assumed that programs are based on maintaining the independence of clients and their informal support networks while providing service to fill gaps without incurring dependence on formal system programs. Examples cited in this chapter are derived from the Continuing Care Program in Manitoba. Many components discussed here will be similar in other programs, but boundaries may be described differently in other programs, requiring different boundary negotiations. In fact, the boundary descriptions have changed in Manitoba over the decade of the program's existence.

Successful programs have a higher ratio of holding cases together than watching them fall apart. A greater proportion of cases will be viewed as satisfying challenges by program staff than as frustrating time and energy consumers. Client service needs will more often be able to be met regardless of whether required services are internal to the program or across program or system boundaries. Relationships of functional reciprocity between systems will be established.

Emerging Long-Term Care Systems

One of the challenges to current program planners is to speculate as accurately as possible on what community-based long-term care programs will look like in the months and years to come. The Manitoba program has experienced changes over time and expects to continue to change as it remains responsive to changing needs of clients, their informal support networks, and the broader community.

Missing services or components of service identified in examples cited in this chapter have become less frequent over the decade of the program and further resource development continues throughout the province. An imperative feature in responding to changing needs is to assure sufficient flexibility of direct service staffing and to maintain adequate program staff (case coordinators, resource developers, and administrative support personnel). Concomitantly, caseloads must be kept at a reasonable size to assure thorough and prompt assessments, regular case reviews, and appropriate reassessments. Also, as more sites for care evolve, community-based long-term care programs will have to be responsive to changing configurations of services necessary to support client independence in these newer settings.

Boundary Issues of the Future

In a milieu of fiscal responsibility and economic constraint, responsiveness to changing client needs will have to be accomplished through redirection of existing resources. This redirection will come either from within these programs or across boundaries within the broader social and health systems. Under these circumstances, boundary negotiations will become even more crucial. In part, because of this anticipation of both more negotiating and more necessary innovative boundary crossing, it will become even more essential to assure adequate program staffing and to maintain sufficient direct service staffing flexibility. If the Manitoba Continuing Care Program has learned one thing through painful experience, it is that there are no savings from curtailing program staffing. Unrealistically large caseloads inhibit prompt assessments, slow down case reviews, mitigate against appropriate and timely reassessments, and preclude innovative solutions at program boundaries. They incur either client dependence through delays in withdrawing unneeded services or increased costs by employing easy solutions. This often means providing more costly services that are integral to the program even if personnel are overskilled for requisite tasks.

In summary, boundaries will likely change over time as will client needs and community resources. However, boundary crossing will remain essential to community-based long-term care programs. Sensitivity to changing boundary descriptions, changing potential client needs and characteristics, awareness of new locally acceptable and available sites for care, and sensitivity to evolving potential resource solutions and financial trade-offs will become even more essential for program staff. Simultaneously important will be trade-offs to the clients, the programs, the broader social and health system, and to the community at large. We would hope that in most cases these greater expectations of staff will provide professionally satisfying challenges rather than energy consuming frustrations.

In any case, we are assured that effective boundary crossing and innovative individualized solutions under changing circumstances with responsible fiscal limitations will be even more time- and energy-consuming in the future. Program staffing patterns must be adequate to this challenge or the "institutionally" easy and more costly decisions will prevail. The challenges to community-based long-term care programs will be to assure program integrity, boundary openness, staff morale, and fiscal responsibility in the face of changing clients, changing program boundaries, changing systems, and changing personnel.

6

Computer Systems and Community-Based Long-Term Care Service Agencies

Joan L. Quinn and David W. Rieck

BACKGROUND

Computer use in community-based long-term care systems is just evolving and currently is used on a limited basis only. Collection of client health and social data, along with service cost data over time, is very unusual, except in selected research and demonstration projects. Staff activity and organizational functions are marginally computerized as well.

In 1976, Triage, a long-term research and demonstration project, began the task of investigating computer hardware and developing software packages to capture organizational and client data. Triage delivers services to older people in a selected seven-town area in Connecticut. Its systems, as well as new programs developed under Triage, were adapted to a statewide home care prototype of Triage after the Triage demonstration ended. The statewide prototype is Connecticut Community Care, Inc. (CCI).

As with Triage, CCI provides case management services directly and provides other services through contracts with specific service providers. These services include nursing, home health aides, homemakers, companions, adult day care, home-delivered meals, choreworkers, transportation, and counseling. With over 200 contracts with agencies and individuals, the thought of a manual system was mind boggling. Gathering data about dates of service, units of services by clients, and by region, would have been a task soon subject to error and frustration.

Because of a targeting of services to chronically disabled older persons, many persons remained on the program with contracted services for several years. Consequently, the program had to not only track client changes over time but service changes as well.

SYSTEM DEVELOPMENT

While developing software for the community-based long-term care system, a systematic approach was taken to establish total data processing needs. First, there was documentation of the future short- and long-term agency goals. These were considered by the administrative and case management staff themselves. Next, all other internal staff were surveyed. Third, contact was made with other agencies who used computers. Last, Triage staff discussed its needs with affiliated consultants and hardware/software vendors. The use of consultants and hardware/software vendors was of some help, but because few computer systems were in place for this type of organization, experienced agency personnel were the "best experts" regarding what systems were necessary and how they could be useful. An army of computer salesmen then appeared ready to sell "just the right equipment" to meet the organization's needs. As stated, most of the hardware and software vendors had not encountered a program such as Triage before the meeting. The time taken in shopping for a computer that would meet the organization's needs was an education for Triage staff as well. "How to Buy a Computer" is not part of the curriculum in any graduate program in the human services arena.

DESIGN CONSIDERATIONS

Because community-based long-term care service systems are funded through a myriad of payers, public and private, fiscal reports to funding sources are an important component of a data system. To generate complex reports on large volumes of clients and provided services, a fairly sophisticated system must be built and be capable of multiple outputs. For example, clients by payment source and by town of origin for a specific time period was a necessary report. This data file had to be interactive with selected client characteristics.

Design considerations in the system must be flexible and responsive to multiple users. As there were many components to be investigated in the program, each with particular staff dedicated to that function, things, at times, became rather hectic, especially when reports were due on the same date. Systems must have online data entry and editing capabilities. By developing an interactive environment, information entered can be retrieved and verified, if necessary, in a timely fashion. Personal computers were not available in great numbers when we started, therefore they were not investigated.

The actual hardware configuration that is used to support the case management function centers around a Hewlett Packard 3000, Series III, Central Processing Unit (C.P.U.), which has the following peripheral equipment attached to it:

- two tape drives (1600 b.p.i. and 800 b.p.i.);
- two 120 disc drives;
- one 600 lines per minute printer;
- one plotter; and,
- thirteen terminals (five of the terminals are located in offices away from the central office's Central Processing Unit and are adapted for telecommunication).

MASTER SYSTEMS

A "full-fledged" community-based long-term care computerized system should have three master systems. These systems should be able to collect client information and record service utilization and costs over time. They must be user-friendly for the case management staff. The systems must interrelate. This can result in cost savings, and deliver necessary data when needed. All three systems are discussed in more detail below.

Client Systems

In order to be able to "target" a "frail elderly population," the first necessary data instrument is a computerized client prescreening tool. Every new client referral is asked questions from the screening instrument. Data captured includes source of referral, reason for referral, self-perception of need, physical and social functioning, caregiver support, and financial information. The prescreening tool looks closely at five client variables: functioning level, age, living arrangment, income, and family or other informal support. The case manager then makes a clinical judgment about the older person's need for case management and other services.

Data gathered at the time of prescreening is used and verified at the time of initial face-to-face assessment by a case manager. For those older persons not eligible for the program, the uniform data collected becomes available to substantiate reasons for non-enrollment. Such data is necessary information when an agency "targets" recipients based on their current status. The organization can always be challenged by individuals who state that they were "entitled" to the program services, but were rejected by it.

Out in the field CCI nurse and social work case managers perform clinical assessments either in the client's home or in hospitals and/or nursing homes using a coded, uniform, and comprehensive computerized assessment. The assessment is entered through a system design using screens. This method was selected as a result of initial communications with the software vendor. Data obtained from each older participant includes sociodemographic data, health, social, and environmental data, family support data, and financial information. A computerized reassessment instrument is used at a minimum of every six months. This activity allows for recording of client changes over time. It is then stored in the computer data base. The data is stored on-line and is kept indefinitely. Because of stipulations in state contracts, data must be stored for a minimum of five to seven years. The system was designed to meet this need.

After a client assessment is completed, a plan of care is developed and implemented using resources from the client, families and other supporters, and agency service providers. This care plan is just being put on line now.

The data base established from the referral, assessment, and reassessment documents performs several tasks. It generates referral sources and characteristics of persons referred to the program. It summarizes referral activity, and provides a client census report by region which includes the number of clients referred by the region and town. The information generated is used by town officials to determine unmet needs of its older constituents, by providers of services to determine volume of need, and by legislators to document the desirability of increased resources for the program. In addition, the organization itself can see from which towns and regions it is drawing most client referrals and where it needs to perform more outreach. It produces an alphabetical list of clients, a numerical list of clients, and a client directory. Finally, it creates a listing of future contact and reassessment dates for case managers to use in their daily functions.

The assessment/reassessment data base contains client sociodemographic characteristics as well as functional measures. These include activities of daily living and instrumental activities of daily living, such as the ability to shop, manage money, and take medications. Mental status as well as other questions are asked. These include areas such as medications taken, the clients' health history, current medical treatment, environmental, and family support questions. Information, without individuals being identified, can be aggregated and used for reporting and analysis. By individualizing and aggregating data about client changes over time, case managers can plan for future services. At the same time we review past client changes. Data then may serve as an important reservoir for use in public policy formulation and research about the changing needs of older persons.

Quality control is sustained by computerized "error reports" generated for each case manager for each variable in the data base. As the organization grew, additional data entry personnel and programmers were hired on an incremental basis. Detailed orientation sessions for all staff regarding the data system was necessary. To some, the computer was a challenge to overcome—to others, it was a "terrifying thing."

Case managers do not interface with the computer system, but data entry people can call up information for them. Case managers, as well as administrative support staff, did not originally "love" the system and just lately—five years later—have decided to peacefully coexist with it.

Reimbursement Systems

An ability to process provider claims for services and to capture client "service use" data mark important adjuncts to the collection of client assessment information. We consider four major areas in a client claims reimbursement system. First, there is a client master file which contains identifying information about the client and includes client eligibility status, the client's location (town), and the case manager assigned to the client.

Second, the provider master file contains each service provider's identity, service dates, and types of services rendered, and the provider's allowable charges.

Third, the account master file contains funding sources, units of service, and charges for service. Data can be aggregated by month, by year to date, by type of service delivered, by funding source, and by service unit.

Fourth, the transaction log contains detailed information for each bill processed and can be used for reporting purposes.

Our claims reimbursement data base contains the names of all contracted providers, each contracted service, and cost for each service type by provider. Each claim sent by a service provider is compared with the master client list to assure that the client is active. This is then compared with the provider master list to be certain that only approved services with the appropriate reimbursement rate are being paid. Information is retained for reporting purposes and generates federal and state required reports as well as provider payment reports. Listings of service utilization by client and a summary of costs and units of service used by client, by region, and by case manager are also available. Checks for vendors of service are generated using the computer's check-writing capability.

Agency Management System

It was determined during the early stages of hardware selection and software package development that the community-based long-term care agency itself could benefit from several management systems. The first one to be developed was a financial data base which contains a general ledger and financial statement reporting package. The software package was custom made. It would have been less expensive to purchase an existing system; however, the custom software allows for more particular reports that were needed to respond to varied funding sources. This system retains all financial data for the agency and it is used for developing reports on a per funding source basis by service region (e.g., how many Medicare dollars in region one).

The system also includes a billing/accounts receivable capability and a check-writing cash disbursement program to more efficiently disburse the agency's funds. The financial system can generate many reports, including consolidated and regional reports: balance sheet, statement of income and expense, general ledger, budget-to-actual statement, and by region and funding source with budget-to-actual income statements. The accounts receivable system is generated by fund, by region, and by client.

A case management activity data base is also generated each month. It records case management time spent in the functions of client assessment, monitoring, and service coordination. Files that record this information are interactive with the billing file and allow for creation of invoices for both clients and third party payers.

Other systems important to long-term care agencies that should be considered along the way are payroll and personnel systems.

DEVELOPMENTAL TIME

Thus far, one would think that purchase of the computer and development of software systems occurs without a "glitch." This was not true. The programs were to be ready within six months, however, fifteen months later they were still being tested and "blowing up." Federal and state agencies that get involved in computer acquisition can take an eternity to approve the request for it, while demanding mountains of documentation in "computerese" which few people understand. Ideally, community agencies would like to have complete and ready "turn key" systems. Realistically, it should be expected that, even with promised "turn key" systems, the key will jam and maybe a new locksmith or two will have to be called.

SUMMARY

It is important to evaluate the needs of community-based long-term care organizations so that multipurpose, useful, and cost efficient systems are developed which benefit clients, professional line workers, agency administrators, and the public and private funding sources of the agency.

With the evolution of computerized data systems in community-based long-term care, one can generate information to meet the reporting, fiscal, and managerial needs of the organization. Data can be used to assist in the clinical and management areas and in research. For example, a case manager/clinician uses data collected to closely monitor care and progress of clients; an administrator determines the number of service units used in a specific time period; and a research and/or policy maker employs data from a large number of clients to test a hypothesis or formulate policy. Systems developed respond to all of the specific needs mentioned above. In addition, data can provide reasonable, comprehensive reports which satisfy increasing demands for clinical documentation, quality assurance, and financial record keeping.

Computer storage of data allows for retrieval of information so that untoward demands are not made on case management staff. If, on a Friday afternoon, a representative of some funding source has to know the number of clients with cardiovascular disease taking a cardiac drug that is a beta blocker, the information comes from an ad hoc computer report, not from case-carrying staff.

A FINAL NOTE

We would like to end with a note about the process of getting a system up and running. If your particular agency is beginning to explore computerization please allow as much time as possible for the developmental process. Anyone who claims your agency can be computerized overnight is just plain wrong. Getting a system up takes an inordinate amount of time. One of the principal reasons it takes so long is the degree of specificity needed by the computer people to design the system and the complexity of the different interests (e.g., clinical, administrative, and evaluative) who will use the system. Part of the start-up time is taken in educating the programmers about what the organization needs in its systems. The rest of the time is involved in getting the organization itself to articulate its needs. A simple example—what to do with text storage—should illustrate this process.

Administrative and research staff probably do not need any text stored in the system while clinical staff may find it useful if some narrative comments appear on printouts about their clients. If text is to be entered, stored, and capable of retrieval, how much text—25 characters, 40 characters, or some of 25 and others of 40? Should there be space provided for all areas or just a selected few? If a selected few, which ones, and who selects them? Associated with these questions are real cost considerations (e.g., all text stored means higher storage costs).

Most of us, in our everyday lives, are very capable of dealing with ambiguities, but computer programs need "yes-no" type answers and specific unchanging "if this, then that" rules. Computers can do a lot but they cannot muddle through. They have to know exactly what you want, how you want it, and how frequently. This means a long iterative process of raising the level of specificity of your wants and decisions about those wants. This process amounts to long and successive meetings between all interested parties and then to testing out the technical feasibility of the specifics.

What we, and other agencies who have gone through this stage, have observed is that underlying all these lengthy discussions about specifications is a consensus-building process. A general agreement is reached through a series of compromises. The end result is not as tidy or optimally efficient as if the system were developed singly for one person's use. But, if done carefully and in good cheer, you will get a system that satisfies everyone's most important needs—after a longer period of time than you would have thought initially.

7

Building Bridges between Hospital and Community: An Organizational Perspective

Chana Zlotnick and Melvin J. Weinstein

INTRODUCTION

This chapter describes a pilot effort of our service delivery site, the Comprehensive Family Care Center (CFCC), in the New York City Department for Aging's Home Care Project (HCP). HCP was a four-site, three-year research and demonstration project which tested a community-based approach of long-term care to a chronically ill, elderly, and homebound Medicare population. Project services were targeted to clients who were slightly above Medicaid eligibility levels with insufficient resources to pay privately for service.

We set up this pilot effort, which operated concurrently with another ongoing CFCC program, in an attempt to place at home a small group of patients on "back-up" status in hospitals awaiting nursing home placement. Backed-up patients no longer require acute care but often remain hospitalized due to a lack of adequate community services. A hospital is reimbursed less than normal inpatient rates for these backed-up patients so hospital administrators were interested in ways to facilitate their timely discharge.

Our primary objective was to determine whether 56 hours of our Project homemaker/personal care service could be used to initially discharge and maintain select backed-up patients in the community. A second objective of this pilot effort was to see whether the hours of care could be reduced once a participant stabilized at home. We agreed to provide up to 56 hours per week of our services to this particular population, which was well above the maximum 20 hours per week provided to our regular clients in our other ongoing program.

COMPREHENSIVE FAMILY CARE CENTER

In June 1981 the Comprehensive Family Care Center (CFCC) became the Bronx host agency participating in the Home Care Project. CFCC was the third of four Project sites selected to deliver services provided to clients through Medicare waivers. These services consisted of client assessment and case management, up to 20 hours per week of homemaker/personal care, transportation, and prescription drugs. Each site provided these services, at any one time, to 100 homebound elderly, 65 years of age and older.

CFCC is a community-based health center affiliated with the Pediatrics Department of the Albert Einstein College of Medicine. It serves all age groups but, prior to its participation as a HCP service delivery site, it had not implemented special programs specifically oriented to elders. Therefore, the initial tasks of our Bronx site were twofold: first, to direct the professional community serving the geriatric population to CFCC as a locus of service; and second, to identify a patient population which would meet HCP guidelines.

INTAKE

Since our site was limited to 100 clients in an area of 62,446 elderly, outreach to potential sources of referral had to be done selectively. CFCC staff decided to accept referrals mainly through local social and health service providers who were most familiar with clients in the community. This was done rather than rely exclusively on fraternal organizations, churches, and synagogues.

Both community-based and hospital-based providers were contacted. Community-based agencies were informed at meetings of local Councils on Aging. These Councils function as coalitions for aging concerns within local Community Boards. CFCC site staff also visited hospital-based providers and presented an overview of the project at meetings of social service and discharge planning units. As referrals were received, the site assessment team, a public health nurse and social worker, assessed all prospective clients in their own homes as required by the project design.

Throughout the course of the pilot, project services quite successfully served as discharge resources for our clients who were hospitalized during the course of the demonstration. The requirement of an initial in-home assessment, however, precluded the acceptance of hospitalized elderly who were not already our clients. Discharge planners were reluctant to release these potentially new clients without the assurance of project service. Discharge planners often expressed frustration at the demonstration's inability to serve as a resource for these patients.

BACKED-UP PATIENTS

Backed-up patients were particularly difficult cases to place for a myriad of other reasons. These included legal complications, such as patients not being competent to handle their own affairs; medical complications, such as patients on a respirator requiring continuous supervision; and social problems such as patients who were living in unsafe environments. As if these difficulties were not enough, they were often compounded by pressures which staff felt to speed up the discharge because of the lower reimbursement rate for these patients paid to hospitals. However, many of these patients would consider home care if the linkage to the community could be made.

THE MISSING LINKS: RESPONSIBILITY AND SERVICES

We learned that one of the important missing links in discharge planning seemed to be that neither the hospital nor the community social worker would assume the burden of responsibility for the actual discharge into the community. Hospital social workers or nurses do not actually see clients or patients in the community and are, in a large sense, planning in darkness. Likewise, hospital procedures and planning process are equally a mystery to community social workers who often do not know when to expect patients and in what condition.

Compounding these discharge complexities is a lack of resources available to both hospital and community social workers. Medicare policy limits numbers of days per hospitalization through its Diagnostic Related Groups (DRGs) as well as the numbers of home health aide hours available posthospitalization. This creates a backdrop for the return of a weakened and helpless patient to the community. A community, on the other hand, may lack adequate housing, housekeeping hours, and even necessary back-up telephone reassurance for homebound patients. This was the case of Mr. Furley, who was hospitalized with a second stroke and was then discharged soon after the utilization review committee found him ready for discharge by Medicare standards. The local Area Agency on Aging was unable to provide housekeeping hours due to their burgeoning caseload. Mr. Furley was left in the care of his niece who was holding a "nine-to-five" job. Consequently Mr. Furley, paralyzed on his right side, was left alone all day unable to adequately toilet or feed himself. An appointment with the social worker from the Area Agency on Aging was two weeks off.

AN ACTION PLAN

At its October 1981 meeting, following a careful review of the back-up problem in New York City, the Project Advisory Committee recommended that staff explore the potential to assist backed-up patients awaiting nursing home placement. We felt that the project might be able to make available its Medicare waiver services as a discharge resource to selected backed-up patients. We also felt that project services could adequately meet ongoing service needs of these patients.

Some initial preparation was necessary. Our site coordinator, along with the assistant project director, met with the directors of social services and discharge planning of local hospitals. They grappled with whether project service could adequately meet the community needs of their backed-up patients. They also had to identify issues which would serve as a basis for the design of our effort. Preliminary discussions clearly indicated a need to bridge the gap between hospital and community in order to facilitate discharge planning.

A proposed design based on these discussions developed which included an increase in project homemaker/personal care from a maximum of 20 hours per week, five days a week service provided to typical project clients to 56 hours, seven days a week service for those backed-up clients to be referred. We also waived the requirement of all in-home assessments by substituting an in-hospital patient and supplemental "environmental assessment" for these potential clients. Agencies providing the site with homemakers were notified of our plans and prepared themselves to provide us with weekend service. We targeted our effort at patients of two hospitals.

One of these facilities, a municipal hospital whose social service staff had already been consulted, had previously opened a floor to their backed-up patients. Here, alongside chronic lung disease patients, resided patients waiting for nursing home placement mainly because of the lack of informal supports. This particular floor seemed a logical place to launch our new effort at providing home care for backed-up clients.

IMPLEMENTATION

Our first client was discharged home on August 20, 1982, following a brief assessment in the hospital. Home environment was checked for safety and accessibility with a local community agency and/or family who had prior knowledge of the client. Provision was made for a home visit by the team prior to discharge. This was necessary if there was no family or agency to provide the sought after information. Under no circumstances would we accept a client unless environmental supports were adequate. During the first five months a total of 14 patients were screened and 11 were brought home with anywhere from 40 to 56 hours of homemaker services spanning a seven-day week. However, staff were able to reduce the hours of service initially prescribed in only one of these cases.

Client home environments ranged from those who lived alone to those who lived with a spouse or children. Client diagnoses included chronic obstructive pulmonary disease (COPD), chronic arthritis, hypertension, strokes, organic mental syndrome, and Parkinson's Disease.

What did our effort do to differentiate it from the normal pattern of discharge planning? Basically our effort bridged the gap between hospital and community. In-hospital visits by assessment teams afforded an opportunity to speak with patients' physicians, therapists, and often family. Liaisons already in place with community agencies did a great deal to ascertain the quality of life individuals would have upon return to the community. Service provided to clients through Medicare waivers offered the necessary additional hours of care. This made the crucial difference between an elongated hospital stay and a trial return to home. Moreover, the team that brought the patient home remained to supervise progress at home. There was always a readily identifiable and responsible party. The following case history illustrates how all this actually worked.

Mr. Martin suffered from severe Parkinson's Disease, chronic heart failure, and organic mental syndrome. He was on back-up status, waiting for nursing home placement, because his wife was reluctant to accept the full burden of his responsibility. With additional services, Mrs. Martin welcomed the opportunity to bring her husband home even though she knew that he would need a great deal of care because he was a large man who required both his wife and homemaker to assist with certain tasks such as transferring and bathing. Mr. Martin was discharged with 56 hours a week of homemaking service which he received for 13 weeks until his death at home. Though his death left his widow understandably upset, she expressed comfort in having spent their last days together in their home.

Not all cases had "happy" endings. Mr. Simpson, 80 years old, suffered from emphysema and COPD, and lived alone in a small apartment. His condition was so severe that he was oxygen-dependent prior to his hospitalization. Although his son and family, who lived in a nearby suburb, asked that he move in with them, Mr. Simpson repeatedly refused in order not to burden them. When Mr. Simpson was first approached by site staff about returning home, he expressed great reluctance and fear about doing so without close informal support.

Following several attempts by staff to encourage Mr. Simpson to do so, he finally agreed to return home with project service. Though project service did not prevent further hospitalizations, it did provide an available discharge resource following his need for acute care.

Mr. Simpson managed at home for ten months, at which time his medical condition rapidly deteriorated. He was rehospitalized for an extended period. In August 1983 he died in the hospital following a two-month wait for a nursing home bed.

SUMMARY

About seven and a half months after this effort commenced we began discharging clients due to the scheduled termination of the

HCP. This effort was, therefore, too short-lived for us to evaluate its full impact in all the areas we were interested in testing.

The linkage between the hospital-based and the community-based team, which we were able to put in place, in combination with the 56 hours of project service, enabled us to discharge ten select backed-up hospitalized patients awaiting nursing home placement. Some clients had "happier" stories than others. Though it might be difficult to label a particular story as successful, we believe that our effort did provide a small group of extremely disabled hospitalized patients, with nothing but pending nursing home placement to which to look forward, with the opportunity to return home and in some cases to be close to loved ones. Who's to say that spending one's last months at home, as in the case of Mr. Martin, is any more or less of a "happy" ending than remaining institutionalized, perhaps for years?

Also, the combination of 56 hours of care per week and the extension of the hospital-based team into the community led to a reduction in the cost of care for this particular client population. Had any of the clients discharged because of this effort remained hospitalized, the cost of their care would have far exceeded the weekly cost to the project, approximately $364 for 56 hours of homemaker/personal care.

The one question that remains unanswered is whether these clients' condition would have sufficiently stabilized over time for us to have reduced the hours of service in more than one case. Had our population been larger and the duration of the effort longer, we would have had more conclusive data.

We believe that little effort has, thus far, gone into a full exploration of the issues which we sought to explore in this essay. The potential of such a program to save money makes a strong case for further study. While it may be presumptuous of us to assume that this effort will lead to such exploration, it is our hope that policymakers will recognize the need for further investigation of this particular area of discharge planning.

8

Interviewing Challenges of the California Senior Survey

Anabel O. Pelham and William F. Clark

INTRODUCTION

While foregoing chapters explore issues in community-based long-term care projects from the experimental or client side, this chapter explores the control group side. We tell the story of collecting data about the control group of poor elderly for California's Multipurpose Senior Services Project.

Although all of these research and demonstration projects have had one kind of control or comparison group or another, very little is reported about the reality of carrying out survey research in this context. Knowledge and advice exists about interviewing, but no one can tell you how to convince an elder to talk over the telephone, or let you into the house, or cooperate to answer questions, or allow you to return for a reassessment. How do you dress, behave, and manage in "rough" neighborhoods? What is a definite mistake on the telephone and what types of identification are convincing? The cumulative practical experiences of 13 research assistants who carried out 4,150 interviews over a three-year period of time provide some answers.

When we undertook the California Senior Survey (CSS) in August of 1980, we thought we understood the nature of the task of survey research and the types of individuals necessary to successfully interview the poor, and probably frail, elderly in a three-year panel study. However, what we know now compared to then is a lot like being a quarterback on Monday morning. Hindsight is of course the best sight and it is for this reason that we tell stories about interviewing that we would have liked to have heard before starting the survey back in 1980.

THE SURVEY AND ITS SAMPLING STRATEGY

Organization

The California Senior Survey (CSS) was the name given to the comparison group for California's Health and Welfare Agency's Multipurpose Senior Services Project (MSSP) and funded by a contract through the California State University and Colleges System, fiscally housed at California State University, Fullerton Foundation. MSSP was a three-year research and demonstration project in long-term care and is currently an ongoing program. CSS interviewed approximately 2,000 elders aged 65 and older receiving Medicaid (Medi-Cal in California). CSS had eight survey sites and four subsamples of "community," "hospitals," "nursing homes," and "targeted community" per site. The subsamples are named according to the location of the initial intake of respondents. This chapter concerns the half of the survey in northern California, located at San Francisco State University, and coordinated by the senior author of this chapter. It included the sites of San Francisco, Oakland, Santa Cruz, and Eureka. It is based on interviews with survey staff as well as their written reports. Generous and candid self-analysis by this surveying staff make this chapter possible. The southern half of the survey was coordinated by Professor David L. Decker, Ph.D., at San Bernardino State College. David's southern group produced an additional 4,687 interviews for a statewide total of 8,837.

An initial organizational start-up problem concerned office space and telephones. Although a representative of the Chancellor's Office assured us that this would not be a problem, we soon found out that the "word" had either not reached or affected the individual campuses where the interviewers would be located. It seems that in a nonprofit, public organization like the university, space is both valuable and scarce. Only after concerted efforts by both the northern and southern coordinators were the office spaces found and the necessary telephones installed. Interestingly enough, library buildings seemed to have the most unoccupied offices.

Community Subsample

Our community subsample was randomly selected from the Medi-Cal Central Identification Files (CID) and came to us in the form of computer printouts with potential names and addresses but with no telephone numbers. How we ultimately obtained telephone numbers for these individuals merits a detective novel but it suffices to say here that we did finally obtain them through the generous cooperation of the Social Security Administration.

Hospital Subsample

Potential hospital participants were "somewhat" randomly selected by hospitals' social service staff, who were recruited for the task and were relatively friendly to the concept of research in long-term care. They were friendly as long as they could also refer patients to become clients to the experimental, service-awarding sites. We use the term "somewhat" randomly since the hospital social service staff had agreed to randomly assign patients but that later comparative statistical analyses showed that hospital staff referred "worse off" cases to the client group and the more functionally able to CSS. These differences had to be taken into account in the comparative analyses of MSSP. Survey staff contacted hospital participants after they had been discharged and allowed to recuperate for a time. Some hospital staff persons were more cooperative and objective than others and during the hospital phase these dynamics had a real impact upon interviewers. For example, some hospital contact persons kept our staff waiting for hours in outer offices; others were not friendly about forwarding names of potential respondents; others turned the task over to secretaries; and, others, moving on to jobs in different hospitals, never passed the responsibility on to their replacements. On the other hand, one hospital allowed us direct computer access to the daily output of admissions records (i.e., the "face" sheets). Statewide, we formed working relationships with approximately 25 hospitals.

Nursing Home Subsample

Nursing home participants were selected by culling through Treatment Authorization Request Forms (TAR's) received by the regional Medi-Cal field offices. The MSSP client nursing home subsample was formed in the same manner by the sites' own staff. TAR's are submitted at the point when an individual seeks placement in a nursing home and requests reimbursement from Medi-Cal. Admission to a nursing home can occur very quickly and a large number of TAR's were telephoned in by physicians. The Medi-Cal field office kept a tally of called in TAR's until written orders were processed. There was great potential for confusing duplications here. For this reason, we quickly learned to assign one, and only one, survey staff person to the "TAR Pits" to select the daily interview pool. The special experience of interviewing nursing home patients is described later in this chapter.

Targeted Community Subsample

Originally, targeted community participants were meant to fill in any gaps in the CSS sampling strategy or provide a balance with MSSP clients. The targeted community eventually served the latter function by attempting to represent frail and at risk individuals who, by the operational definition of high health care costs, suggested an increased probability of low functioning abilities. Attempts to locate and interview these individuals were an abysmal failure. The procedure that we used to find these individuals was to first do an analysis of statewide Medi-Cal expenditures. From this analysis we produced a listing of names, ranked in terms of highest expenditures and the most aged. We then proceeded to call these individuals and screen them over the telephone. The telephone screen was to determine if they were low functioning as scored by the Activities of Daily Living Index (Katz et al., 1963). Like others who have gone before us in survey research, we were reminded that the individuals who are the most frail are truly the most difficult to locate. In our case we ran into two specific problems. The first one dealt with our master list of names from the Medi-Cal analysis. We found that the bills containing the expenditures are processed as they are paid. This meant that the actual services had been provided up to six months in the past. By the time we actually called these individuals they had already died or been institutionalized.

The second problem was related to the index we chose to screen the individuals. We found that the Activities of Daily Living Index was, for our purposes, too gross a measure of functioning and that it was not discriminating enough. It seems that individuals either possess all or most of the functioning abilities of this Index or they do not possess any of them (i.e., they are dead).

If we had to do this task again we probably would use the same type of Medi-Cal analysis, acknowledging its time limitations, but use another screening instrument which would be more discriminating. An index that comes to mind for this purpose is the Instrumental Activities of Daily Living (Lawton and Brody, 1969).

The participants that we did find for the targeted community subsample turned out to be the frailest subsample of the entire client and comparison group sample, but we only filled about 15 percent of this subsample before we finally stopped trying.

TRAINING AND SUPERVISION

The CSS interview instrument's length and coding complexities necessitated thorough initial interviewer training and statewide staff education sessions following the two major revisions and updates of the questionnaire. Statewide training also served the latent functions of providing a reality test for the instrument developers, affording an opportunity for interviewers to learn about the "big picture" from state level staff, and, finally, offering a public forum for concerns, questions, suggestions, and complaints about interviewing. We found that the strategy of interviewer training where trainees would score along with a videotaped interview of an elder and a walk through the instrument item by item was invaluable in catching and quashing ambiguities before they could become candidates for instant, but ephemeral, operational definitions. It was also during the second round of interviewer training that we were reminded of the critical necessity of having an on-site supervisor. If the interviewers have only to pick up the telephone or come across campus to fix a scheduling inequity; settle a quality control debate; return the call of a worried daughter about the interview of her mother; offer another operational definition of incontinence; call about a late paycheck; or just "talk it over," the survey runs much more smoothly indeed.

INTERVIEWER CHARACTERISTICS

Because of funding regulations and the structure of the California State University and Colleges system, we were obliged to confine our potential staff recruiting pool to CSUC students and affiliates. Recruiting was not open to the general public.

This was acceptable, as years of experience teaching field work courses in gerontology had produced a fairly clear notion of qualities to be sought in student interviewers to be hired. This experience had taught that gerontology students who were to survive the rigors of participant observation and remain analytical had to possess a number of special characteristics. We soon labeled this persona a kind of functional schizophrenic, split between empathetic and analytic. Unfortunately, literature describing the ideal survey interviewer was ambiguous and of little help.

At the height of its staffing levels, northern California interviewers consisted of 13 individuals: three males and ten females, and ages ranged from the middle 20's to the 40's. Ethnic groups represented included Blacks, Chinese, Japanese, and Caucasians. Four staff persons were multilingual and seven were graduate or postgraduate students.

Gender

Interviewer age or ethnic status appeared to have no effect on being well received as an interviewer. Gender did, however, have a negative effect if the participant was a nervous elderly female and the interviewer male. This was easily resolved over the telephone by substituting a female staff person.

Physical and Psychological Health

We learned that our interviewers needed to be fundamentally healthy and in even better physical condition than the average individual. Learning the intricacies of a 50-page instrument, becoming immersed in a subculture of the poor elderly, and undertaking the task of a relatively lengthy interview took a toll on the health of the staff. Although we do not directly correlate staff illnesses solely with the task of interviewing, as some interviewers were also graduate students and holding down other positions, we do believe that there was a significant amount of stress that was job-related and may have affected health status.

Over the duration of the survey our staff experienced almost chronic upper respiratory infections, one broken ankle, two accidents requiring hospitalization, two gynecological infections requiring hospitalization, one fractured knee, and assorted depressions. The requirement for physical health became so important that when the Santa Cruz interviewer left the survey to enter graduate school we replaced him with a qualified woman who happened to be an athlete. Her status as a marathon runner, touring cyclist, licensed scuba diver, and hiker caught our attention and her resume rose like cream to the top of the pile of job hopefuls. Carol of Santa Cruz, by the way, suffered no illnesses.

Becoming "stressed-out" as an interviewer was common. Staff persons had windshields broken, tires flattened, and cars towed away. Staff were bitten by dogs, threatened and pushed around by street punks, and had guns pointed at them. While in participants' hotel rooms, staff were propositioned by prostitutes who teased while nude in doorways; observed heroin use; were yelled at by others in the household; had roaches drop from the ceiling into their hair; and had mice scurry across their feet. One female staff person even contracted a case of scabies. These occurrences were not everyday but their cumulative effects created such ambivalence that one of our most dedicated interviewers confessed, "I'll be glad when this is over."

The requirement for mental and emotional health also became painfully apparent as the stress of interviewing poor, ill, and often depressed elders began to accumulate. High stress periods usually followed any kind of change, such as change in coding the instrument, a revision of the instrument, traveling into a different area of town, and particularly moving into a new subsample phase (e.g., from community to hospital to nursing home). These adjustments were usually followed by an increase in what we came to call "Walks around Creative Arts." That is, when staff persons became upset, angry, or depressed about the effects of the task, we would leave the confines of our fluorescent box of an office and take a walk around the Creative Arts Building and look at the trees and flowers and talk it over.

Can You Live with Uncertainty and Ambivalence?

An alteration in instrumentation or a new subsample phase also generated a rash of "what if" questions. That is, interviewers needed clarifications and interpretations of the letter and spirit of questions. During such transitional stages, the survey coordinator became the on-the-spot, instant articulator of operational definitions—like it or not. For example, when one received a frantic telephone call at 4:30 on Friday afternoon asking what if a participant used a three-legged cane with wheels—was this to be coded independent in ambulation or not? Thus was born an operational definition to be renegotiated on Monday morning and communicated to all interviewers up and down the state.

Anticipating the human factor and breakdown in communications associated with ad hoc operational definitions, a heroic effort was undertaken by a designated research associate to maintain high interrater reliability among interviewers scattered from Eureka, near the Oregon border, to San Diego, adjacent to Mexico. The investment was successful as CSS staff usually scored in the middle to high 90's in reliability tests (Scherf, 1982 and 1983).

Perhaps most critical to interviewer success and survival in a three-year panel study of the poor elderly is a philosophy of life that allows the individual to live with uncertainty and ambivalence. This includes everything from debating an instrument coding question for two days to watching a beloved participant suffer and die following a stroke. In an almost Darwinian sense, interviewer success and survival depends largely upon an ability to quickly adapt to a problematic reality. "Can you live with uncertainty and ambivalence?" became a central question that we posed to prospective interviewers during the second round of hiring.

Attention to Detail

The final product of the survey was a machine-readable interview. Since the questionnaires were all key punched the interviewers had to be careful about simple things such as neatness and legibility. We instituted quality control measures at the local offices where interviewers would "QC" the questionnaires of other interviewers. Peer pressure had an amazing effect on the overall quality.

However, being overly scrupulous about neatness had its disadvantages. In the last year of the survey we discovered that we were missing the questionnaires of interviews that we knew had been done. Upon a little discreet investigation we found that a few interviewers had "hoarded" the forms until they could make them perfectly neat. It turned out that the "hoarders" were also the perfectionists when it came to quality control. Fortunately, we retrieved these forms and no harm was done. A little perfectionism goes a long way.

Desirable Interviewer Qualities

By the second round of interviewer hiring, approximately a year into the survey, we felt we had a sense of at least some of the qualities that make up a good interviewer.

They are:

- good physical and emotional health, including a sense of humor and perspective;
- the independence to schedule assigned interviews, with access to an automobile, and to follow specific detailed instructions without constant supervision;
- a personality that allows for early rapport in human relations;
- a clear understanding of the "big picture" and mission of the research such that one is not moved to "split frog hairs" to answer a question; and,
- a genuine humaneness and respect for the dignity of others and a concern for the elderly.

STRATEGIES THAT DID AND DID NOT WORK ON THE TRAIL OF THE FRAIL

Getting the First Interview

Some staff felt that the most difficult part of the job was in the beginning, getting the initial interview. Most requests for interviews were done over the telephone, and quite naturally, people were suspicious at first. It took a lot of cajoling, prodding, and convincing to set up the interview. If staff thought the elder lived with family it was helpful to offer to explain the project to another in the household. Sending printed information about the survey prior to the initial telephone call had mixed reviews. Sometimes it helped, sometimes it made no difference. We suspected that many potential participants living in residence hotels never did receive our correspondence.

During initial telephone contact, staff quickly learned by trial and error not to ask for Ms., Mrs., Miss, or Mr. anything. Potential participants with unisex names like Willie Jones took instant offense if you got their gender wrong. It also instantly identified you as an outsider. During initial telephone calls, staff found that use of the word "survey" was counterproductive. Staff quickly abandoned a carefully constructed telephone script to employ their own easier, more natural, and successful "party line." Interviewers identified themselves as representing the Health and Welfare Agency, not the California Senior Survey. The former had unquestionably more positive impact.

For the most part, we have found the more ill a person is, the less likely s/he is to consent to an interview. Staff have sometimes been able to talk a person into the interview by assuring her/him they would stop as soon as s/he got tired and would finish the next day, or whenever they were feeling better. At other times, the $15 stipend paid to participants per interview was the deciding factor. Our assessment of the value of a $15 stipend is mixed. To some individuals money was a great influence, to others none. The checks did, however, remind participants of who we were and added to our credibility.

Survey credibility problems were much more prevalent in large cities. Public service announcements on the radio and advertisements in local and senior center papers about the research project had little impact. Seniors did not get the word. We are not aware of one case where an elder learned about the CSS from the media.

Our early reception in Oakland was so dismal that we appealed to a friendly minister for a letter of support from the Mayor. Mailed and hand-carried photocopies of the Mayor's letter as a form of identification had more effect than reams of assurances from the State and all the powers of the fourth estate.

Overall it has been difficult to convince potential respondents that the survey is "on the up and up." They have heard so often about people who prey on seniors that they are suspicious of anyone calling and asking to come into their homes. They thought the $15 was just a line to convince them to agree to open their door to a stranger. Since the most suspicious were adamant, we had little success in changing their attitudes.

A few times we had people refuse interviews because they were going to have to answer personal questions. Again, they seemed to feel that the information was going to be used against them, perhaps to decrease their benefits. Our attempts to assure them this would not be the case were successful some of the time. However, when cutbacks did occur in Medicaid (Medi-Cal) benefits, caused by a statewide budget crisis, our credibility took a severe beating, phone calls poured into the university, and staff became the objects of significant amounts of anger, frustration, and questioning.

Whether over the telephone or in person, if a staff person could explain to a potential participant that a long range goal of the CSS was to keep people out of nursing homes the elder was very likely to respond positively. Also, if the interviewer could convince the elder that they were in no way connected to the Medicaid (Medi-Cal) program per se it was all for the good.

When potential participants did refuse an initial interview, staff felt that reasons were almost always related to fear—regardless of the explanation stated on the telephone or at the front door.

Another telephone technique that took a long time to learn by trial and error emerged in Oakland. We discovered that if a woman answered the telephone, staff should immediately explain the purpose of the call rather than ask to speak with a male participant or elder family member. Women at home during the day were apparently gatekeepers of household business and would routinely deny that person X was at home when we thought otherwise. This was particularly true for women staff persons calling for male participants.

Once the elder agreed to be interviewed, appointments tended to be made during school hours to avoid gangs or punks in rough neighborhoods. This strategy also became automatic in unfamiliar neighborhoods in Oakland.

Even though we experienced substantial difficulty in obtaining that first interview, subsequent analyses of the Medi-Cal expenditures of our respondents showed that there was no statistically significant difference between the mean Medi-Cal expenditure of our respondents as compared to the statewide mean Medi-Cal expenditures of the 65-year old and over age group ($p. \leq 0.05$). There was, however, a statistically significant difference in the variance. Given our experiences in trying to persuade the most ill to participate, this piece of quantitative data did not surprise us.

UP TO AND PAST THE DOOR

Appointments for interviews were best made one or two days in advance. Some elders had a tendency to forget you were coming if, for example, you set up an appointment a week ahead of time. Staff became adept at anticipating the rhythm of the postal service, and in timing reminder letters to arrive shortly before scheduled appointments, and in calling right before the meeting on the day of the interview. Morning seemed to be better for interviews. People were more alert and therefore able to answer a long set of questions in one session.

No staff person could afford to be a clotheshorse but clothing worn on interviews did have some unanticipated influences. Skirts and heels worn in San Francisco's Tenderloin were a problem for women staff as they tended to make one look like a social worker and attract street punks. Male staff also discovered that a more casual dress was less intimidating than a coat and tie. It seems that the desired persona is that of a kind of hip community worker, at least in cities like Oakland and San Francisco.

Most interviewers adopted the habit of carrying a briefcase or valise of some sort for questionnaires and forms. Staff soon realized that briefcases carried around housing projects served as props and were part of the costume of social workers. Because "workers" were welcome in the housing projects where we worked, interviewers acquired briefcases and began to "pass" as social workers.

Parking problems, including parking tickets and being towed away, for interviewers were chronic. Stopping at an empty spot across from a recreation center cost one staff person a broken windshield. Another had her tires flattened.

A few initial interviews were held in public places like coffeeshops or at the university at the request of participants. Usually by second interviews, staff were invited to private residences.

We found that printed individual business cards were extremely valuable in providing credibility and a convenient way for participants to locate us. Interviewers had the option to have their home telephone numbers printed on business cards and many opted to do so.

Once interviewers got past the threshold there emerged the task of establishing rapport. Staff reported that if first direct contact was made with the elder her/himself the dialogue would proceed more smoothly than if they were intercepted by a son or daughter. Patient explanations were always provided but time consuming for interviewers paid on a per assessment basis.[1]

[1] In 1983 staff received $58 for an initial assessment and $32 for a reinterview. They also earned a base salary of $564 per month for office and survey related tasks. During the Fiscal Year 1982–1983, the total cost per interview, excluding data processing, was $170.

During early minutes of initial interviews we found that a good way to "break the ice" was to inquire about pictures of family or other items on display around the house.

One young female interviewer learned early on her first assessment not to suppose what an individual's race might be. Our interviewer guessed wrong about the category and the participant was furious! Fortunately there was no harm done and this "wisdom" was passed along at the next staff meeting.

Interviewers usually engaged in a fair amount of physical contact with participants. Handshakes were the norm.

Face to Face Problems

Government People. Problems during interviews were varied. Many people had difficulty comprehending the purpose of the interview, but often were willing to go along with it anyway. They seemed to lump all "government people" together into a generally powerful and threatening group who should be obeyed. Although about 25 percent of the participants were suspicious of our intentions at first, most were secure after a relatively short time. Recent immigrants were particularly vulnerable to such "government people" assumptions, especially Russian Jews. However, once they realized that we were no threat to them, their attitudes changed. They were so grateful to be in the United States and with an American that their adoration was embarrassing. It was a constant struggle for staff to explain the benign nature of their visit and our sincere wish for truth through a mouthful of baklava.

Relatives. Relatives were one of our most consistent and frustrating complications of interviewing. Even after a pause to explain that the interview was explicitly for, say, their mother, they would often continue to interrupt, correct, or criticize the respondent's answers; sometimes, it seemed, affecting the honesty of subsequent responses.

Families can go either way in acceptance of survey research. Some will insist on being present or will not care to get involved. For longitudinal studies, it is best to find out family preferences at the first interview. In some cases, families can be major, dependable, and accurate sources of information.

Mental Status. Interviewers quickly learned it was important to get an immediate sense of the respondent's mental status before coding an hour and a half's worth of hallucinations. Staff persons observed that the mental status questions per se did not necessarily reflect a "functional" mental state. Interviewers found that people "know what they have to know" in order to get along with their particular social context. For example, it is not important for a 90-year-old woman living in a lovely loft in the family Victorian to know "the name of the President of the United States before this one."

If interviewers suspected that the intellectual functioning of a participant was impaired the rule was to "patchwork" together an assessment employing as many helpful informational bases as possible (e.g., home helpers, family, or head nurses). But even with the "patchwork" methodology there was a sincere commitment to obtain as much information as humanly possible from participants. Staff began to employ particular questions in the early sections of the instrument as "tests" of intellectual functioning. "What was your principle form of employment?" and "Where were you born?" seemed to lend themselves to this purpose.

Finding the Common Ground. Inside residences, some interviewers found that personal attention makes a difference. Some staff found that talking about problems that an elder parent or grandparent had experienced with Medicaid (Medi-Cal in California) indicated that you were not part of the system. Other staff attempted to locate other "common grounds" of experience. One male staff person interviewing in Oakland discovered that he shared the pastime of betting on horseracing at Golden Gate Fields. Sharing horseracing and betting experiences helped a lot.

Food. Food offerings became a standard social anemity during—but usually before—interviews, and in some circumstances interviewers also had silent mental questions about sanitary conditions. No one became seriously ill but some staff complained of gaining weight. Some participants went to a great deal of effort to bake homemade ethnic pastry and native dishes. With Russians and Filipinos one is invited to eat pastry and/or fruit. On interviews with Samoans one is expected to stay for a lunch feast.

Food was also a useful tool for interviewers. A staff person had one female participant who suffered depressions and tended not to want to see anybody during these periods. On more than one occasion she responded positively when told that the interviewer was looking forward to coming over for some of the delicious tea she brewed.

Troublesome Questions. During actual interviews, deviations from training tended to take the pattern of interpreting a sometimes "intellectual" section for participants or softening the impact of emotionally-charged questions. For example, many elders were not knowledgeable regarding medical terms and commonsense words had to be substituted for medical conditions. We experienced this same difficulty in reverse with interviewers. They knew what a medical condition and its general symptoms was—but were unfamiliar with treatment therapies, drugs, and common or slang terminologies. A registered nurse who was working as an interviewer developed a concise dictionary of medical conditions as a reference for the staff.

A proportion of participants did not want to answer particular sets of questions on the instrument. The Cornell Medical Index, Mental Status, and Life Satisfaction questions were the worst offenders. Some participants called these "dumb" and refused to answer. These respondents explained that the questions did not make sense. Interviewers picked up on the negative attitude and began to turn it around with the preface, "I know this may sound silly, but I have to ask it anyway." This humble approach usually satisfied reluctant respondents and the interviews would proceed.

Some questions on the interview were very personal and staff found it valuable to ask each question as if it were important but not to press participants into answering. This can result in falsified information concerning such questions as, "How many friends do you have?" It is hard for some people to admit that they have no friends, overdue bills, emotional illness, or grooming problems. Sometimes when participants were in critical trouble (e.g., following an amputation), staff found difficult questions hard to ask and interpret. Life Satisfaction and Mental Health indices were particularly awkward during life crises. On the other hand, participants would go out of their way to answer a question. One participant called an interviewer at 8 p.m. at home to tell her excitedly that she had just remembered the past President of the United States!

Because interviewers were instructed to code as "per self-report," problems associated with second guessing were eliminated. However, the questions of truth and accuracy had to be addressed. We desired the truth, of course, but whose truth and whose reality?

Communication Problems. In cases where participants could not communicate very well, but were not intellectually impaired, interviewers would offer a "word salad," that is, guess at the list of responses and seek a confirmation. This approach was particularly useful with stroke victims. A signal with the hand was a common form of confirmation.

Interviewers recount that hearing problems were a constant challenge. Communicating with a nearly deaf person is exhausting. Participants sometimes become impatient, accusing interviewers of talking too fast or mumbling. There was no easy solution to this problem. In the beginning, we assumed a hearing aid would make life easier for everyone—the respondent, as well as for relatives who seemed to have given up trying to communicate with or include the senior in their conversations and activities. But too many have told us about their experiences with hearing aids that buzz, do not fit properly, or—and this appears to be the most common complaint—simply amplify garbled voices. On more than one occasion staff noticed that people who were described by their children and grandchildren as being senile were actually hard of hearing. They were responding to questions the way they heard them—which was often incorrectly. Accordingly, their answers appeared to be nonsensical. However, if the same question was repeated very loudly and slowly, participants answered quickly and correctly. Although the relatives were aware of the hearing problem, they did not realize how it affected communication.

Hearing problems could also be a source of humor, especially to seniors themselves. An interviewer remembers that, "When I asked one man if he was a bedwetter, he replied, 'That's why I moved out here, because of the bad weather.' When I repeated the question (more loudly), he laughed as hard as I did."

Regarding functional ability, staff had to occasionally remind themselves that one ages differently and therefore will make different demands of the interviewer. As one interviewer recalled, "A mistake I once made was to almost shout the first few questions at one respondent who had no hearing disabilities. I had just come from an interview where the person was just about deaf. Needless to say the respondent cringed at my loud voice."

When participants were non-English speaking and staff did not speak the language, we found that employing the same interpreter was particularly helpful in overcoming awkwardness. In regard to translated assessments, we found that it was better not to schedule two in the same day because it was difficult to coordinate six schedules in one day (the interviewer's twice, two respondents, and two translators).

Even if a participant spoke English, a certain amount of translation and interpretation was often necessary. For example, the "laundromat" became the "washhouse" and "monotonous" meant "boring." "Breaks in life" was translated as "good luck" and "maiden name" became "mother's last name before married." "Immunizations" was interpreted as the familiar "flu shots" and "dreary" was "unhappy." Interviewers explained that "on top of the world" meant "very happy" and "down in the dumps" did not mean literally spending time at the sanitary landfill.

Focusing. Once a decision was made to participate in the interview process, there was no problem in getting people to talk; the problem was trying to get them to stop. Or at least to limit their responses to when their sister last wrote (as opposed to ". . . she was never worth two cents, you know, let me tell you about the time she. . . .").

Time spent during the interview process created a fair amount of dissonance for staff persons. On the one hand, interviewers explained that it was important to know how to stop conversation, otherwise you could spend hours at each interview. On the other hand, there was the guilt felt in not being able to spend more time socially with some of the people who had so little social interaction in their lives. Some participants worked at making interviewers feel guilty and were quite successful.

Staff described interviewing as a constant balancing act between being businesslike and efficient and being friendly and sensitive. The success of one demeanor over the other is dependent upon the respondent. Some respondents just want to answer the questions, with no chitchat. Others must be almost "courted"—with a cup of coffee, "how are the children?," "nice weather we've been having"—before the interview. If these courtesies were not extended, participants were offended and let you know it. In general, people were reasonable about sticking to the questions. They were usually respectful of an interviewer's time and knew that they were there to do a job.

Getting Ready for the Next Time. Even before the first interview ended, staff prepared to locate the participant for the next assessment. From hard experience, we found that the most effective, almost failsafe, strategy, was to identify two contact persons, preferably two who lived outside the participant's household. It saved a lot of time when trying to track down a "lost soul." Staff also discovered that sending a personal letter in a personal envelope helped to find people and get a response.

Reassessment Problems

Reassessment problems were not as multiple as on initial interviews but they did possess some unique characteristics. For example, quite a few of the respondents forgot from one interview to the next who the staff were and what the survey was all about. This resulted in one staff person being thought of as psychic when she asked about a poodle. The participant thought it was her first visit. Before going on a reassessment, we found it useful to check in with the last interviewer to visit the participant before making an appointment to learn the idiosyncrasies of the participant's family or environment. We also found that it was better not to switch interviewers for reassessments. If a switch did occur, the "new" interviewer often ended up telling the participant all the latest news about the other interviewer.

Also, it was sometimes helpful to make a couple of notes on what was going on in the respondent's life (e.g., an expected trip) during the initial interview. Then when calling to reschedule, some personal interest can be shown (e.g., "How was your trip?"). This helped insure a more cordial reception for the interviewer, and reduced refusal rates. Finally, when calling the participant on the telephone for a reinterview, recalling the last interview and who you were was helpful, as was mentioning the check that CSS sent them.

On a positive note, interviewers observed that hospital subsample participants were often significantly improved by the first reassessment. On a negative note, staff often felt helpless in the face of overwhelming cumulative injustice. One female interviewer explained that it was difficult to know what to say to people who say time after time that they have nothing more to live for and are ready to die, or that they have no one else "in their right mind" in their nursing home or board and care home who they can talk to or spend time with. Boredom was described again and again to be a major problem of the seniors who were mentally active, but physically frail and socially isolated. During the survey we received a telephone call from the coroner's office attempting to identify one of our participants. The only personal document he had on his body was the $15 honorarium check from the California Senior Survey.

Friendships. During the three years of the survey most interviewers became friendly with participants and some developed full-time close contacts with frail elders. Such elders had interviewers as their only major contact and the participant became emotionally dependent because of the intimate knowledge and because the interviewers cared. Most interviewers who formed friendships with the aged felt that if you allowed someone to be emotionally dependent on you, you must assume that responsibility of following through with being their friend.

Gifts. Occasionally, little gifts as tokens of friendship were exchanged between participants and interviewers. Participants would bake or sew a little handmade gift and staff would bring a toilet article like bath powder. We did not encourage gift exchange but it was impossible to stop, particularly gifts brought to patients in nursing homes. The Northern Coordinator herself had been soundly scolded by the friend of a Tenderloin hotel resident for not accepting an old fur hat. The friend had to remind the Coordinator of the larger functions of gift exchange in human groups. Our rule for expensive gifts, however, was to decline and, if pressed, make a little joke about leaving it in the will.

Humor. Regarding joking, one interviewer argued that, "I don't think most people realize how anxious seniors are to laugh. Most of them have open minds and love a good joke." For example, one interviewer said, "The wife of one respondent refers to me as his 'girlfriend' when I come to see him. She always asks if we want to be left alone. I tell her I'd rather she stay in the room, because I don't trust him. Seniors are very often terribly funny. They are candid about me ('I liked your hair better the other way.' 'Why aren't you married?'), grandchildren ('spoiled brats'), and of course politicians (obscenities)."

Keeping Track. Keeping track of who was due for a reassessment was, initially, an administrative recordkeeping problem which took months to iron out. Looking back now, we should have invested more time in the beginning to design a reassessment schedule that was operative from the start. Another procedure which we should have instituted was to have the interviewers file a report each time a reassessment was missed. A report like this could assist finding those "lost souls" through queries to the local Social Security Administration office and, if unsuccessful, the county's office of Vital Statistics could be queried to determine if the respondent had died. We did institute such search procedures on an ad hoc basis at the State level and interviewers developed their own strategies (e.g., reading the obituary column in the newspaper) but, on reflection, a more formal set of procedures probably would have been more useful.

The Special Case of Nursing Homes and Culture Shock

Regardless of planning and good intentions, learning to cope with nursing homes and patients was, again, largely by trial and error —the hard way. None of the interviewers had previous experience with nursing homes and our explanations did little to diminish the trauma of culture shock. We could not prepare them for the "weirdness" of the experience. This problem was more serious than we realized, particularly for the staff person doing most of the assessments in one large county home.

For nursing home patients intellectually intact and otherwise, many interviewers found it useless to make appointments. Our staff would drop by during visiting hours. However, on the initial nursing home visit, interviewers would first go to the administrator and if s/he was unavailable go to the director of nursing or head nurse instead. Nurses in charge would usually allow access to patients but not to records and it was at this point that interviewers were referred or bounced back to administrators.

Generally speaking, nursing homes were less than enthusiastic about our visits. They were concerned about evaluation, insurance, outsiders, and any other number of reasons to deny access. Once inside nursing homes, interviewers quickly learned not to show up between the hours of 11:00 a.m. and 1:00 p.m. so as to avoid waiting around while the patient eats lunch.

When calling ahead was desirable or advised, interviewers learned a kind of telephone assertiveness. They simply informed the director of nursing that they were coming and inquired about the best time. Interviewers learned that if they asked to come, they were routinely told "no" or told "yes" by the director of nursing but who also referred them back to the administrator who did not return calls and, after a go around, said "no." An administrator's denial reopened the renegotiation process from the university office and this was repeated almost every time that there was a turnover in nursing home administrators or directors of nursing.

Individual staff business cards were particularly useful in the nursing home phase. Interviewers were routinely asked to show several forms of identification and, for this reason and to create a familiar presence, we made an effort to assign the same staff person to a particular nursing home. Our "nonthreatening familiar presence" strategy seemed to be successful over time and interviewers became part of the background scenery.

When nursing staff were called upon to assist in a proxy interview we found that they were more likely to agree if assured that the $15 stipend would go directly to the patient for his/her personal needs and not into some controlled account. Obviously, we could assure that stipend checks would be made out to the individual nursing home patient, but we had no control over who managed the money.

Interestingly, we learned that wearing formal clothes was helpful in nursing home interviews—particularly initial ones. Our one male Caucasian interviewer was almost always assumed to be a physician and called "Doctor" when on a nursing home interview. None of the women or ethnic minority male staff were mistaken for physicians.

Aside from the actual interview itself, staff explain that recording the medicines that people were taking from medical charts and obtaining this information was the hardest part of the task. Sometimes medication information was denied to interviewers and they had to ask nurses to verify certain data. Under such circumstances staff learned that making nurses feel important, valuable, and helpful was a good idea. Eventually, we dropped this section from the questionnaire and obtained medication data directly from the Medi-Cal expenditure computer tapes.

Staff believed that medications and drugs create another kind of problem for them in nursing homes. It appears that patients who were the most intellectually and emotionally impaired were also the ones who were taking the most drugs and combinations of drugs. It was a real problem keeping drugged patients on track.

Staff observed that approximately 15 percent of their nursing home participants were severely intellectually impaired. In addition, hearing problems were very common. Adaptive modes like speaking slowly, clearly, and loudly, showing the questionnaire, sitting by a good ear, and sign language were helpful, but were not cure-alls.

Clearly, the nursing home subsample phase was the most difficult and emotionally traumatic for CSS staff. They had to learn to get used to nursing homes with odors, filth, illness, and tragic human conditions. Our interviewer working in the county home returned to the university office twice in shock after visiting locked wards and a coma ward where individuals had been wired to life support systems for an average of four years each. We found it advisable, because of the stress, not to schedule two nursing home assessments in the same day. It was simply too exhausting.

Regardless of our subsample site or phase, interviewers attempted to give to our elders a sense that they were making an important contribution to a statewide study of long-term care and that their individual efforts were valued and appreciated.

CODA

When we began the California Senior Survey in August of 1980, we had no idea of how hard it was to contact the frail elderly or the nature of the difficulties involved in obtaining access to acute care hospitals. We did not know how interdependent we would have to become, or how many different work roles we would come to assume. We could not guess then that we would need to make time to laugh and cry together—if only for a few minutes around the photocopy machine.

In many ways, the California Senior Survey has been a lot like a mission. We joked to ease the tension about being "on the trail of the frail." Now that the survey research has ended we have learned a great deal about the interviewers as well as the interviewed.

We know that our staff have become friends with some participants and unofficial social workers in some desperate cases. We discovered that a staff person told a lie about a 100-year-old participant's functioning ability in order to help her get accepted into a social service project. One interviewer admitted to helping a wheelchair-bound participant escape to a different floor of the county nursing home for some privacy with his new bride—also confined to a wheelchair. We learned that a quiet champagne dinner was planned by an interviewer for the last assessment with a special participant. We have been told of an idea of one of our bilingual interviewers to introduce all her lonely Spanish-speaking participants to each other.

We have been reminded that our interviewers are very special people themselves—in their humanity and humaneness—and that they forged close relationships with each other. In many ways the survey staff became like family and like all families the breaking up was difficult when the survey was completed.

REFERENCES

Katz, S., et al. Studies of illness in the aged. *Journal of American Medical Association*, 1963, *185*, 914-919.

Lawton, M. P., & Brody, E. M. Assessment of older people: Self-maintaining and instrumental activities of daily living. *Gerontologist*, 1969, *9*, 168-186.

Scherf, B. A. Interrater reliability: Initial assessment instruments. California Multipurpose Senior Services Project, California Health and Welfare Agency, Sacramento, Calif., 1982.

Scherf, B. A. Interrater reliability: Revised assessment instruments. California Multipurpose Senior Services Project, California Health and Welfare Agency, Sacramento, Calif., 1983.

9

Project Termination: Reintegration of Demonstration Clients into Existing Service Systems

Melvin J. Weinstein and Chana Zlotnick

INTRODUCTION

A major concern to staff of any time-limited, social intervention research and demonstration project is the discharge of clients at the study's conclusion. A project usually provides services to participants for a designated period and then terminates. These services are often unavailable outside of the demonstration. When participants are vulnerable and at risk, concerns about client well-being due to the termination of project services are further heightened.

This chapter describes the process of planning for and actually carrying out the reintegration of demonstration clients into the existing service delivery systems due to the termination of New York City's Department for the Aging's Home Care Project. The Home Care Project (HCP) was a three-year research and demonstration project which operated from mid-December 1980 through March 1984. HCP's staff provided case management services to project clients, as well as arranged for homemaker/personal services and transportation services, and paid for prescription drugs not normally reimbursed by Medicare.

HCP's host agency, the Department for the Aging (DFTA), is a public agency concerned with delivery of service to the nearly 1.3 million New Yorkers 60 years of age and older. DFTA is also the designated Area Agency on Aging and is responsible for administering a broad range of services including congregate and home-delivered meals, employment, and homemaking.

HCP itself had a centralized staff located at DFTA and four

service delivery sites in select neighborhoods of New York City. Two of these sites were health-related and two were oriented to social services.

DFTA sought Medicare funds from the Health Care Financing Administration (HCFA) and special funds from the Administration on Aging (AOA) to test a community-based approach to long-term care for the chronically ill, elderly homebound, and Medicare population. These elders were slightly above Medicaid income eligibility levels but with insufficient resources to pay privately for service. The basic motivating idea behind the demonstration was to show that this community-based approach would enable this population to remain at home rather than be placed in nursing homes. While preparing the initial application for HCFA, DFTA staff gave considerable thought to what would happen to clients after this time-limited demonstration was over. In the beginning, staff felt that the traditional services available in New York City, such as home-delivered meals and Title IIIB homecare services, would sufficiently meet the ongoing needs of most clients at the project's conclusion.

Unexpectedly, the project enrolled a much more disabled population than anticipated, and their needs could not be met with these traditional services. This necessitated unanticipated planning during the course of the project. It also necessitated extensions of the project service periods beyond the original termination date. These extensions enabled staff to fully explore a variety of new resources available after termination which could best meet the actual needs of the 400 frail participants. In some cases, these participants had received comprehensive services for over three years.

Issues discussed in this chapter include planning for project termination; identification of discharge resources; negotiation for referral agreements; and the realities of actually carrying out client discharge. We end the chapter with a discussion of our experiences and our recommendations for this painful process.

PLANNING FOR PROJECT TERMINATION AND CLIENT DISCHARGE

DFTA started planning for the reintegration of project clients at the conclusion of the demonstration during the initial grant preparation. During the start up phase, DFTA submitted a plan to

HCFA which had made release of initial grant funds contingent upon submission of a satisfactory plan to wind down the demonstration. Of most concern to both DFTA and HCFA was the adequacy of existing community resources to be used to meet the ongoing service needs of project participants at the demonstration's conclusion.

Subsequent to the submission and approval of this plan by HCFA we did not readdress discharge planning issues until a year before service termination was to occur. At that time, with one year to go, the project and site staff realized that available service resources would fall far short of meeting the needs of most project participants. This belated realization, to a large extent, was due to the fact that actual project enrollees were significantly more disabled than the population initially targeted for services. For example, except for those clients eligible for Medicaid benefits, resources in the preliminary plan offered only limited amounts of homemaking service. These amounts were well below the 20 hours per week of homemaker/personal care that many participants received through the demonstration.

During the course of the final year, administrative and case-carrying staff frequently met to develop a strategy to address the issue of alternate service inadequacy. They subsequently developed a Client Discharge/Project Termination Plan that would form the basis for winding down the demonstration.

Among issues immediately identified was the need to locate suitable resources available upon discharge to meet the high disability levels of clients, particularly for the estimated 250 who remained eligible for only Medicare benefits. For those clients who had become eligible for Medicaid during the course of the demonstration, a wider range of services were available through that program. We also needed to update staff knowledge of recent changes in entitlement policy. In addition, we had to negotiate a special policy for the expeditious handling of project clients' applications for Medicaid benefits. Finally, we wanted to develop a suitable time schedule for the entire discharge process.

Feelings of disappointment, depression, and fear on the part of clients and staff confounded these issues. Even though they were informed from the beginning about project termination, clients felt disappointed that the project, which had so ably provided for them in the past, could not continue. Staff, aware of their accomplishments with these clients over the last several years, felt frustrated with the paucity of alternatives available at discharge. As one case manager stated, "First we're the good guys and now we're the bad guys."

As a result of the planning meetings, staff developed a discharge timetable. A cutoff for accepting new clients was scheduled to occur six months prior to termination of site operations. Client discharge was to occur during the final three months of service delivery.

In the intervening months, the schedule was revised three times. Two revisions came about because HCFA extended the project's operating authority and the third was due to our own planning purposes.

The first change was made when HCFA approved a three-month extension of the project's operating authority. Although this extension had been approved solely for research purposes—to permit the collection of a minimum of a full year of data on all clients—it also had the effect of extending the availability of services.

Administrative and case-carrying staff met to consider the implications for the clients. We agreed to move back the date of discharge to coincide with the new service termination date. We also agreed to extend the discharge period from three to six months.

The decision to extend the discharge phase was made for four reasons. First, we recognized the need for additional time to plan for the discharge of those clients for whom available services appeared to be inadequate. Second, there were, as there still are, the difficulties in New York of accessing skilled-level nursing home beds from the community. Third, we had to take into consideration the anticipated reduction in sites' capabilities to manage ongoing workloads due to staff resignations. Fourth, and finally, we were not sure of clients' reactions who had been informed and prepared for the earlier termination date.

The second change occurred approximately four months later after HCFA approved an additional six-month extension through March 1984. HCFA approved this second extension to provide staff with additional time to continue to identify and to develop new alternative services for the clients who were most difficult to place.

The third revision was made by administrative staff several weeks later, following a review of the progress of the discharge process. This final change moved the date of service termination back from March 31 to February 15. This revision was made to permit a minimum of a month and a half of follow-up with all clients, particularly those whom we judged would have the most difficult postproject adjustment problems. This change was also due to administrative concerns about the number of staff who would be available at each site, at that time, to care for clients.

While these extensions and changes ultimately enabled staff to successfully discharge and place nearly all clients, these changes also affected the discharge process itself. We discuss the impact of these changes in the section, "Carrying Out Client Discharge."

Concurrently with development of the Client Discharge Plan described above, we developed training sessions to update staff knowledge about recent changes in entitlement policies. Additionally, we developed special procedures for handling and processing project client applications for Medicaid and Medicare homecare benefits. Also, DFTA, HCP, and site staff sought to identify and negotiate referral agreements with potential resources at the time of discharge.

IDENTIFICATION OF DISCHARGE RESOURCES

One of the primary tasks facing staff was identification and development of suitable discharge options for clients. This need for adequate discharge resources was the principal factor leading to a reexamination of the original wind-down plan. This process jointly involved project and site staff. The local sites focused on local community-based services while HCP central staff sought potential opportunities available through citywide and statewide sources.

To assist in this process, we surveyed site staff and asked them to evaluate their caseloads and to explore potential arrangements for their clients (e.g., nursing home placement, Medicaid eligibility, community services, or private pay options). Although we knew that client populations at each site would change somewhat from the time of the survey to actual termination, the survey results provided staff with an initial guide to the type, level, and amount of service for which planning would be needed.

One finding of this survey was the unexpectedly large number of clients who, during the course of the demonstration, had become eligible for Medicaid. Medicaid benefits in New York State are quite comprehensive. From the perspective of arranging for services after termination, this turn of events was quite helpful.

For example, Mrs. Thomas, who lived by herself in a tiny bungalow in an obscure section of one site's area, experienced a decline in health status during the course of the project. She had also become eligible for Medicaid. When Mrs. Thomas was first admitted to the project she was approved for 12 hours per week of homecare services. As the project was terminating, she was accepted into the Medicaid Homecare Program and scheduled to receive seven hours a day, seven days a week service.

Another example during the discharge process was Mr. Frank. Site staff recommended that he "spend down" to become eligible for Medicaid and its broader range of services. In this context, "spend down" means that an individual divests him or herself of property or income or other assets to meet the means test of the Medicaid program. In short, one becomes poor on purpose. Mr. Frank not only suffered from peripheral vascular disease and chronic heart disease but also experienced a significant increase in need while on the project. Although Mr. Frank agreed to follow staff recommendations, his wife resisted due to her concern about being left alone on Medicaid without financial resources of her own. The couple's family agreed with Mrs. Frank and Mr. Frank was finally discharged with insufficient care.

The stressful ethical dilemmas which this story typifies raises serious questions. Is Mr. Frank better off with the prescribed services which could be obtained by becoming "poor on purpose" or in the care of a proud and caring but clinically unskilled wife without recourse to needed professional services? It is a sad commentary on the times that such questions are even raised and sadder still that they have to be answered and resolved in the last years of life.

Nonetheless, the discharge process continued and project staff requested special meetings with New York City's Medicaid Homecare administrative staff to seek a cooperative agreement for transfer of clients. These meetings led to development of special procedures to expedite processing of applications and for implementation of services to our clients applying for benefits. These procedures included a simplified application review process, designation of staff to be involved in the effort, and the establishment of a communications link between site and Medicaid staff.

On the community level, site staff negotiated referral agreements with local agencies participating as service delivery sites in the New York State Long-Term Home Health Care Program (Lombardi Program). This program is designed to provide comprehensive community care to eligible Medicaid recipients.

Despite these developments, staff continued to be most concerned about those project clients who remained eligible for only Medicare benefits and for whom adequate community services were not available. Nevertheless, site staff began to meet and negotiate agreements with providers of available community service, including home-delivered meals, Title IIIB homecare, and church-sponsored volunteer programs such as "friendly visiting." These community services could be used in the event that additional alternate sources of service could neither be located nor developed. In many cases, staff found themselves negotiating referral agreements with the very same agencies who had referred their most disabled clients to the sites at the beginning of the demonstration!

Several problems immediately arose in the process of developing these agreements. First, the local agencies themselves were quite reluctant to accept back clients who, in the first place, they were unable to serve and who may have deteriorated even further during the demonstration. For example, Mrs. McKey was referred to the project by a community agency and suffered a stroke while she was our client. This stroke left her even more disabled. Efforts at negotiating for her return to this particular agency at the project's conclusion were not successful. Ultimately, Mrs. McKey was placed in a nursing home.

Second, many agencies expressed reluctance about giving project clients priority for services ahead of persons already on their waiting lists.

Third, some agencies felt that the Department for the Aging (DFTA) should provide increased financial support to better enable them to absorb and service our project's clients.

Reintegration was more problematic for the project's two hospital sites. Both hospitals had to rely solely on outside local organizations as referral sources since neither ran programs which could meet the in-home service needs of chronically impaired clients. In contrast, the two social service sites were in a relatively better position to offer some ongoing services through existing programs under their auspices. However, neither of these social agencies could provide the high level of services comparable to that received by clients through the project. These factors led to a more intense exploration of alternative discharge resources.

NEGOTIATION FOR A COMPREHENSIVE REFERRAL AGREEMENT

After exploring resources on a client by agency basis, project staff began negotiations with DFTA's Public Works Program (PWP), a program which provides homemaker service to non-Medicaid, homebound elderly. The idea was to match our referrals with Public Assistance (PA) recipients who are required to work a designated number of hours each week to maintain their PA eligibility. This program offered the most potential as a resource for the project's Medicare population since PWP could provide ongoing service. Furthermore, the effort had support of DFTA's executive staff and negotiation of a comprehensive agreement would presumably be more easily accomplished since PWP was also a unit within DFTA. However, there were several obstacles involved in the PWP program which required special attention. Of most concern was the fact that PWP provided a maximum of six and one-half hours per week of only homemaker service. This was far below the 17 hours per week average of both homemaker and personal care services received by project clients.

Although we realized that a replication of project service would not be possible, DFTA was most interested in providing services to clients which, as much as possible, matched services received through the project. A review of PWP led to a plan to increase the service offered from the six and one-half hours per week of homemaking service normally provided to a maximum of 15½ hours per week of homemaker/personal care services for referred project clients.

To increase the level of service and to ensure effective care to a population much more highly impaired than that typically served by PWP, several program modifications were made. First, to ensure a core group of reliable and effective workers, it was agreed to recruit personnel by requesting volunteers for the effort from among those workers already in PWP. Second, it was agreed to increase the amount and the level of training provided workers from 40 to 90 hours and to gear additional training to personal care tasks. Third, DFTA committed funds to employ a full-time public health nurse to train and supervise the workers who would participate in this effort. DFTA also agreed to retain appropriate project staff, beyond termination of grant funds, to continue to work closely with service site staff to coordinate the transfer of demonstration clients to PWP.

To further ensure success, the four project service delivery sites were permitted control over personnel issues such as hiring, placement, and retention of workers. Additionally, a plan was developed for the eventual transfer of these clients to other local agencies to ensure clients a continuity of service.

Concurrently with the development of the PWP alternative, staff pursued other options. These included Section 2176 Medicaid waivers, Emergency Jobs Bill resources, and Community Development 9 funds.

Although planning for the discharge of the Medicaid clients was well underway when the discharge phase formally began, staff realized that additional time would be required to fully explore all options for the Medicare-only clients who were inappropriate to spend down to Medicaid.

Consequently, DFTA executive staff requested a one-year extension of the Medicare waiver services. The request was made following a review of the remaining population and time requirements for a thorough exploration of all remaining service opportunities and for discharge of clients. About six weeks following DFTA's request, HCFA approved a six-month extension.

During the following three and one-half months we made the above mentioned modifications to PWP and it was geared up to accept our referrals. We also fully investigated other options. None were found to be feasible, due either to time constraints or to the limited availability of funding in New York City.

CARRYING OUT CLIENT DISCHARGE

All clients were initially informed about the time-limited nature of service delivery in the project's consent form, which they were required to sign upon entering the demonstration. Not surprisingly, clients and families often denied this reality despite the fact that they were reminded by site staff about the limited duration of the service.

During routine home visits by site staff, when eight months of services remained, clients were formally reminded about the project ending. As previously described, during our last year the termination date of service delivery changed several times. While these extensions provided staff with the time necessary to develop the most effective discharge resources, the resultant changes affected the discharge process in several ways.

In a few cases, the extensions exacerbated the denial syndrome and confused clients even further about the date of termination. This frequently led to a diminution of staff's ability to effectively work with clients. This was the case with Mr. Dalton. As Mr. Dalton was informed about each new extension, he began to doubt the credibility of staff, whom he felt were becoming increasingly deceptive. As a result, Mr. Dalton became less cooperative and more resistant to working with staff around realistic discharge planning. Unfortunately, this led to a less than satisfactory discharge, both in terms of feelings and adequacy of arrangement.

Project and site staff were, therefore, particularly sensitive about the need to communicate information about these changes without exacerbating denial, confusion, and resistance among those clients ready for discharge. In general, staff avoided mentioning the changes in the termination dates to clients but rather mentioned only that some additional time to plan for discharge would be available if needed.

In a number of cases the extensions did enable staff to spread out discharge over a period of months, which was helpful with some clients such as Mr. and Mrs. Lawerence. Mrs. Lawerence was 84 years old and suffered from Alzheimer's disease and Mr. Lawerence was 87 and had severe arthritis. The couple had a difficult marriage and staff, on occasion, had evidence that Mrs. Lawerence had been beaten by her husband, who was overwhelmed by his wife's condition. In addition, the couple were estranged from their two sons.

After repeated staff efforts at involving the two sons in discharge planning had failed, staff recommended placing Mrs. Lawerence in a nursing home. Mr. Lawerence began the process of applying for Medicaid but refused efforts to place his wife. He similarly refused to consider placement with his wife. As an interim measure, the site's social worker was able to enroll Mrs. Lawerence in a local daycare program. This separation lessened the burden on Mr. Lawerence and gave Mrs. Lawerence the structured environment she needed. These efforts took place over a six-month period. Mrs. Lawerence was eventually placed in a nursing home, with Mr. Lawerence receiving homemaking assistance in his own home.

Some participants benefited because the extensions provided staff with the time necessary to seek out and combine resources which most adequately met total client need.

This was the case with 80-year-old Mrs. Bretschneider who lived with her 83-year-old husband in a local housing project. In addition to arthritis and severe hypertension Mrs. Bretschneider experienced difficulty in getting about her apartment as a result of a stroke which she had suffered several years earlier. During this time, increased anxiety and frustration experienced by Mr. Bretschneider in caring for his wife led to a recurrence of an old drinking problem.

As termination approached, the Bretschneiders were advised to apply for Medicaid because of Mrs. Bretschneider's excessive need for services and other multiple problems within the family. The processing of their Medicaid applications dragged on over an extended period of time due to the unavailability of several pieces of required documentation. The extensions enabled staff to continue to provide support and assistance to the Bretschneiders throughout the duration of these negotiations and to implement a package of services once Medicaid was in place. This package included homemaking and twice weekly visits to a local adult day care center. At this center Mrs. Bretschneider received physical therapy and socialization services. These visits also provided desperately needed respite for Mr. Bretschneider.

In at least one case the extensions negatively affected other areas of family life. This was the case with our client Mrs. Gallagher, who lived at home with her husband and their adult mentally retarded son. The extensions led Mrs. Gallagher to believe that the project, on which she so heavily relied, would continue indefinitely and that her husband and son would eventually be enrolled. Her belief that her son would be provided project service interfered with and delayed the efforts of her son's social worker to secure a sheltered workshop placement.

DISCHARGE PATTERNS AND PRIORITIES

Discharge Sequence

One basic similarity to emerge among sites during the termination phase was the order in which discharge planning was initiated with clients. To a large extent, this was related to the anticipated difficulties in arranging for alternate services. In general, discharge planning was first initiated with those cases thought to be the easiest to plan for and sequentially progressed to the most difficult clients.

Among client characteristics used by staff to evaluate potential ease of discharge were the availability of financial resources, availability of informal caregivers, and ongoing service needs. Discharge planning was often first initiated with those clients for whom clearcut service options were available (e.g., participants who had become eligible for Medicaid benefits). Similarly, those less impaired clients who were able to have their needs met privately or with informal help were discharged first.

Sites subsequently initiated planning with those clients whose service options might have been considered by staff to be equally as clearcut but who would possibly require considerable counseling. This second group included clients recommended for Medicaid spend down and clients in need of nursing home placement.

The most difficult group of clients to plan for, and therefore the group with whom discharge planning was often initiated last, were Medicare-only eligible elders, whose needs could neither be met through informal help nor existing community services. Nearly half of the total active caseload at that time fit into this category.

Frequent Change

A second similarity to emerge among sites was the frequent change in client circumstances which necessitated changes in a discharge plan. Site staff often found themselves shifting focus midstream with clients in preparing for discharge due either to a change in health status, death of a spouse, disclosure of new information, and/or refusal of clients to accept recommended service options. Most typically, sudden deterioration of health status and revelation, by clients, of previously concealed financial resources often required alteration of discharge plans.

Client Refusal

Perhaps the most frustrating pattern for sites were those clients who refused to accept the resources recommended by staff. Client resistance and refusal, always frustrating and difficult issues, were even more so because of the pressures of termination. Many of these clients rejected services subsequent to an investment of considerable time and effort by staff. Clients in this group were among those to be discharged last and often with the least satisfactory service arrangements in relation to need.

For example, Mr. Catanzaro, 94 years old, lived with his second wife whom he brought over from Italy. Partially blind, suffering from organic mental syndrome and chronic heart disease requiring a pacemaker, Mr. Catanzaro was also a resistant individual. His wife, whose English was extremely limited, was very concerned but was unable to provide assistance to Mr. Catanzaro due to a hernia condition, in addition to her own advanced age. They refused nursing home placement despite the strong urging of Mr. Catanzaro's son. Homemaking services under Medicaid were proposed but Mr. Catanzaro's son did not wish his father and stepmother to pay into the program. At the time of discharge, there were no known arrangements for homemaker or any application for Medicaid assistance.

Family Meetings

One of the primary objectives of site staff throughout this period was the engagement of clients and families in the discharge process. Staff were familiar enough with most cases that tentative plans were usually developed and then shared with those who would be involved in decisionmaking. Discussion about discharge often took place with clients long before formal discharge meetings occurred. These formal meetings were usually held with clients to discuss the various options being recommended by staff and to formalize discharge plans. In many cases, therefore, these discharge planning meetings merely formalized arrangements previously discussed with clients and families.

TERMINATION PROCEDURES

After discharge plan agreement, staff continued to work closely with clients to arrange for alternate services. During this period staff and clients were usually in close contact about developmental status of plans and clients' concerns and fears about termination.

Once plans were in place, clients were informed and given a date when they would be discharged from the project and transferred to alternate service. Discharge occurred on the day that the primary service project-provided homemaker/personal care was terminated. In nearly all cases, termination of all three project services—homemaker/personal care, transportation, and prescription drugs—was concurrent. However, we provided for clients with significant hardship, such as those requiring thrice-weekly dialysis, to receive transportation and drugs for a short time after termination of homemaker/personal care.

As much as possible, site staff attempted to arrange for transition meetings, usually involving themselves and new service providers, in the homes of clients, on the day of discharge. These meetings provided staff with an opportunity to say goodbye to clients and to oversee transfers of responsibility.

As one can imagine, some of these meetings were very stressful. For example, Mrs. Berry, who had lost her entire family during World War II, became very attached to her social worker, who happened to speak her native language. While on the project, this ease in communication was particularly comforting to Mrs. Berry. At the project's conclusion, her parting with her "friend" the social worker was particularly difficult and painful.

Provision was made for a maximum two-week overlap period between the project and new homemaking service if it was felt that such an arrangement would ease a transfer of responsibility. While this provision was rarely implemented, it was usually done to orient the new homemaker.

Following termination, site staff usually maintained contact with clients for a brief period to monitor adjustment. Most frequently, follow-up involved one or two telephone contacts with a client subsequent to their discharge.

ARRANGEMENTS FOR DISCHARGED CLIENTS

At the end of the discharge phase, all remaining 342 clients had been discharged. We met the deadline which we had set for ourselves. The largest single group, 23 percent, was incorporated in the PWP Homecare Program and only seven percent were placed in nursing homes. Approximately 90 percent of the clients stayed in their own homes. This high rate of success made the efforts to arrange alternative services very worthwhile and satisfying.

TERMINATION ISSUES

This chapter described the process of discharging participants due to the termination of the New York City Department for the Aging's Home Care Project. This was a most difficult and trying time for staff and clients. It was also a period when a number of issues, faced by staff of any time-limited, social intervention research and demonstration project, were clearly brought into focus.

The resolution of these issues can easily be postponed until they arise as crises during final months of operation. Our hope is that this discussion will prompt those involved in similar efforts to give discharge planning the time and attention we now believe it deserves. The four major issues are: (1) service comparability; (2) planning for client discharge; (3) scheduling for client discharge; and, (4) unpredictability in client discharge.

Service Comparability

Services provided project clients are usually unavailable outside of the demonstration. This was the unfortunate reality that Home Care Project staff faced as they began discharge planning with clients. Except for those clients discharged to Medicaid and to private care, most participants were discharged with services well below levels received through the project. At best, staff were able to arrange for a mix of service, such as PWP and Title IIIB Homecare. This service package was offered to those Medicare clients with the greatest level of need who chose to remain in the community. Unfortunately, the opportunity for staff to combine services as often as they might have liked was greatly reduced by the limited availability of alternate services in relation to total client need.

Lack of comparability between project and alternate existing services should be reviewed with staff early in a demonstration. This will also encourage staff to be alert to potential opportunities for services which they may hear about during the course of a demonstration. It will also enable staff to more effectively and realistically discuss discharge plans with clients whenever the issue arises without raising any false expectations. These options may require considerable time for development as was the case with PWP. Raising issues of comparability early in the project may make the difference in staff ability to fully explore and develop options in time for client discharge.

Planning for Client Discharge

Planning for client discharge should be an ongoing process involving both administration, staff, and clients. The process should begin as early as the initial staff orientation and continue throughout the project's duration. A preliminary discharge plan should be drafted shortly after operations begin. This plan should subsequently be reviewed by staff and administration at scheduled intervals.

Scheduled and frequent reviews should enable early identification of any limitations that may arise with the plan due to unexpected circumstances. This process should also foster the timely development and implementation of corrective measures.

The Home Care Project enrolled a significantly more disabled population than anticipated. The project's preliminary discharge plan addressed needs of the "anticipated" population. Fortunately, limitations of the plan that arose due to this discrepancy eventually were realized by staff so that additional discharge options, such as PWP, could be explored. Though modifications to the plan were made, these modifications required additional time which project staff was able to secure from HCFA. Had a formal review process been scheduled, it is quite possible that these same modifications could have been made during the routine course of the demonstration without the accompanying disruptions to staff and clients caused by the extension of service delivery.

Scheduling for Client Discharge

Amounts of time which a project will require to transfer clients from demonstration services to alternate existing services will depend on at least three factors. First, the anticipated time which will be required to gain access to alternate services. Second, the time needed to work through client issues such as denial, resistance, and refusal to accept discharge options. Third, external circumstances may affect staff ability to discharge clients.

To calculate service accessibility, staff should consider both the anticipated time to implement alternate service as well as any problems that can arise during processing which may result in delay. For example, New York State Law requires the processing of Medicaid applications within 30 days. However, during the processing of client applications, Home Care Project site staff frequently encountered difficulties, such as the lack of supporting documentation and the inadvertent submissions of incomplete applications. This frequently led to delays of up to four months before Medicaid could make a final decision.

Secondly, staff should also make allowances for time needed to work through a variety of client issues such as denial and resistance. This should be anticipated and can cause even further delays in client discharge. Most typically, clients applying either for nursing home or to Medicaid offered site staff considerable resistance before applying for benefits. Unfortunately, staff were not able to counsel clients and pursue benefits concurrently since client resistance often had to be worked through before they would even agree to apply.

Thirdly, external circumstances will arise during a termination phase which will hamper staff ability to discharge clients. Project staff initially planned for a three-month client discharge period. This was later increased to six months following a review of a number of concerns including the anticipated gradual reduction in site capability to handle discharge due to an increase in staff resignations toward termination of site operations. Such circumstances can often be anticipated and should be considered by those involved in developing a schedule for client discharge.

Unpredictability in Client Discharge

Finally, some issues will arise during client discharge which will either be unpredictable, or if predictable, difficult to anticipate. For example, during early planning stages for termination, Home Care Project staff recognized the need to provide for follow-up with all clients subsequent to their discharge. Although discharged clients were no longer considered active cases, we felt the need and responsibility to follow up with all clients to monitor their immediate adjustments to alternative services and to be available to them if we felt that our intervention would help. As a result, provision was made in discharge plans for a period of follow-up with all clients. In reality, when follow-up occurred, it usually involved one or two postdischarge telephone calls to monitor client adjustment to alternate services.

On occasion, however, staff dealt with cases where the length of follow-up became the critical factor in determining the date of discharge. This situation most frequently arose when clients persistently refused to accept discharge resources being offered by staff. Most often this involved clients being referred to Medicaid due to excessive service needs.

Whenever staff encountered such cases they were faced with the painful dilemma of how best to reduce client resistance. Should service and counseling continue to be provided concurrently, in which case a client might be left at the end without service and professional support; or, should the client be discharged with the expectation that service deprivation would reduce resistance in sufficient time for staff to provide assistance to obtain benefits during follow-up?

Cases such as these, which fortunately arose infrequently, required a thorough evaluation by site staff as well as flexibility to plan the most advantageous arrangement. While a rigid policy directing the handling of such cases would have been unrealistic and impractical, the availability of a general project discharge policy was critical in guiding staff through the discharge and termination phases of the Home Care Project. Equally critical was the teamwork involving both administration and staff in developing that plan and the kinds of alternative services which could, as much as possible, best meet the ongoing needs of clients at the project's conclusion.

ONE FINAL NOTE

Our final note deals with the practicality of limiting HCFA-funded demonstration projects to three years. Termination concerns dominated our energies during our last year. We spent almost an equal amount of time in the beginning to start up and fully implement the project. This left approximately one year of "demonstration." Given the realities of start-up and termination, limiting projects to three years does not adequately allow for the measurement of observed effects. Three years do not allow enough time for the demonstration to demonstrate itself.

10

Social Policy Implications of the Community-Based Long-Term Care Experiences

William F. Clark and Anabel O. Pelham

. . . this sad blind alley which God has made of old age.

Mimnermos, 600 B.C.

INTRODUCTION

Alternatives do exist to the potential "sad blind alley . . . of old age." However, a common theme running through these chapters is that change does not come easily. In this chapter we define the problems of long-term care. We then offer some alternatives and evaluate them according to our specified criteria. These alternatives incorporate lessons learned from experiences of our contributors. Our specific policy proposals should facilitate change and increase alternatives available to the elderly.

SOCIAL CONSTRUCTION OF PROBLEMS

A major policy stumbling block in the way of reforming long-term care is that no consensual definition of problems exists. To illustrate, we hypothesize problem definitions from different points of view.

- "I'm fine, I just don't want to die in a nursing home. A little more money wouldn't hurt." (The "typical" elder)
- "I need more funds, more flexibility, and more control over the docs." (The "typical" community-based long-term care agency administrator)

- "I need higher reimbursement rates and less paperwork." (A "typical" nursing home administrator)
- "I need less government regulation, less paperwork, and better reimbursement rates." (The "typical" physician)
- "We need information." (The "typical" gerontologist-social scientist)
- "We need to limit expenditures." (The "typical" government fiscal person)
- "We need to help the elderly." (The "typical" legislator)

These are fictitious statements but we have all heard them. Some common themes emerge from the declarations. First, personal and professional autonomy is highly valued. Secondly, most parties see the need for more resources. Thirdly, governmental decisionmakers presently view the need to limit social welfare expenditures. Finally, while the elderly have widespread political support, special interest groups involved in long-term care (e.g., physicians) make up powerful political constituencies. Each of these themes merit special attention. We believe that they make up the constitutive elements of our problem definition.

These themes can be restated in a more general framework. That is, when creating social policy and its subset, social welfare policy, three fundamental questions must be posed. What is the problem? (Keeping in mind that there may not be one, that others disagree about the problem's nature, or that you defined it incorrectly.) Who has the problem? (Keeping in mind that you are labeling a group deviant and they may neither have the problem nor appreciate your interference.) What to do? (Keeping in mind that "help" is almost always defined from the point of view of the more powerful helper, that help is never without cost to the giver and receiver, only the medium of exchange is different, and that institutional empires have been built while undertaking the burden of helping.)

While it is not the intent of this chapter to undertake a phenomenological exploration of the social construction of aging, it should suffice to say that this is our orientation. We do not believe that the phenomenon of aging is solely a biological given with prespecified social consequences. Existing social consequences have come about not because of some preordained order. Aging does not exist independently of our definitions and resources. Consequences are the accumulation of past and present human decisions. They have been socially constructed. As such, present policy repertoires are malleable.

What makes policy creation in the area of aging particularly difficult is that the constitutive elements of the problem definition tend to be at opposite ends of the particular continuum in question. For example, along the autonomy continuum, personal autonomy is potentially conflictive with professional autonomy. The case of Mrs. Reilly in Chapter 4, in which the woman wanted to return directly home from the hospital and her physician wanted a nursing home placement for her, exemplifies this conflict. Also, as Chapter 4 tells us, the elder without an advocate often loses this battle.

Along the resource continuum, the issue of funds is another conflict area. Practitioners need more and government fiscal officials want to allocate less.

Politics are inherently conflictive. How does the typical legislator balance the interests of the elderly consumer with the provider interests, for example, of the American Medical Association, which spent $50 million in its opposition to the passage of Medicare (Harris, 1966)?

These conflictive areas are only illustrative of this turbulent policy area. Conflicts also exist within practitioners' groups as to the best way to deliver services and what those services should be.

No doubt these conflicts rage in other areas such as mental health or child welfare. One basic difference between other areas and long-term care policy is the amount of public funds involved. Depending on how you count and who is doing the counting, we are talking about close to a third of a trillion dollars! This includes Social Security benefits, Medicare, Medicaid, social services, Veterans Administration, the Older Americans Act, subsidized housing, and food stamps. Medicare and the elderly's share of Medicaid and social services programs totaled nearly $100 billion in 1983. As we discuss our major themes of autonomy, resources, and politics, the magnitude of the public dollars and stakes involved should be kept well in mind.

AUTONOMY

Personal Autonomy

In many ways, aging in America represents accumulated losses in personal autonomy. Like concentric circles created by a pebble tossed into a placid lake—only in reverse—aging too often represents a progressive shrinking of the social world. As social roles run a life cycle or are eliminated, their concomitant professional and social networks evaporate. Chronic illnesses associated with very advanced age can turn a benign or manageable environment into a world of unintelligible garble, dim images, unappetizing meals, unsure footing, drugs, sharp edges, and forced solitude. If emotional stress and mental illness are indeed associated with a feeling of helplessness and loss of self control, it is not surprising that for many the later years are extremely problematic. Yet, as a physician who would rather make house calls explains in Chapter 1, relatively minor interventions can reverse a closing circle of old age. Applied holistic geriatric health care, with advice as simple as "remove those pesky area rugs," can have an enormous impact on everyday life.

Aging social policy is shaped by politics, politics are affected by ideology, and ideology is a product of assumptions about the nature of mankind and the social positions of interest groups.

In America, personal autonomy is a valued ideal. Social systems are created and organized based upon assumptions of independent social actors in human groups—except where the aged are concerned.

The problems of the aged are largely socially constructed and based upon the notion that there is an equivalence between aging and dependency. Personal autonomy, like liberty, requires constant vigilance and if it is the nature of the human beast to suffer diminished vigor with advanced age then the maintenance of personal liberty will require social support.

Autonomy, as a concept, may also be employed as an explanatory tool to explore the problems of professionals in caring for the aged: the problems of professional autonomy.

Professional Autonomy

In their attempts to function independently according to professional goals and objectives, health and human services workers often find themselves on a collision course with stated and felt needs of the very elders they are attempting to serve. We have observed the "counter-elder" situation occur because of the nature of a particular position; because of a position's relationship to a larger institution; and because of dynamics among and between professional groups (Pelham and Clark, 1982).

Even so-called public servants can become adversaries, as the social workers in Chapter 2 realized. When faced with the task of combating the existing system to get a snow plow into an inner city neighborhood to rescue a homebound client, they had to behave as a bureaucratic guerrilla team.

During our study of hospital discharge and placement decisions we found multiple examples of professional activities running counter to either the wishes or the continued autonomous status of an elder patient. In the case of discharge planners, we find that they almost always opt for a patient's discharge to home whenever humanly possible. However, caseloads are often enormous, time is short (discharge planners are often among the last to know about an impending discharge), and alternatives are few. As a result, discharge planners frequently find themselves scrambling around looking for a suitable nursing home rather than putting together a service package that would have allowed the elder to return home.

Overseeing this discharge process are the regulatory utilization reviewers. Before the era of Diagnostically Related Groups (DRGs), the main weapons of utilization reviewers were the clock and calendar. As soon as a Medicare or Medicaid patient was certified as nonacute, reimbursement to a hospital moved to a lower level of payment or ceased. Now, with the DRGs for Medicare patients, length of stay is linked to a prospectively paid admission diagnosis. In such cases, hospital discharge planners charged with the task of coordinating a complex discharge and/or placement find themselves potentially at odds with hospital administrators who are loathe to absorb the costs of needy patients, and utilization reviewers who disapprove such expenditures when time runs out.

An elder patient with nowhere to go may find him/herself discharged to the street.

Even if institutional pressures do not force an untimely discharge and/or undesired placement, ultraprofessional competition and conflict over turf can easily shuffle a less than aggressive elder into a nursing home. Just as matter tends to disorder in nature, frail elders tend to be at risk of being placed in nursing homes unless heroic efforts are undertaken to counteract this tendency.

We have observed situations in hospitals not unlike the classic scene in a whodunit film where the lights go out, you hear a scramble in the darkness, and the thief escapes with the jewels!

Only in our case, the lost jewel is an elder patient rolled out on a gurney to the nursing home while physicians, nurses, Medicaid and Medicare reviewers, social workers, discharge planners, and administrators attempt to function autonomously—all in the best interests of the patient.

Although high quality patient care may be the first priority of medical professionals, there are other agenda items as well. Physicians, for example, are looking for bed turnover, unless the patient presents an interesting case. Because the aged typically suffer from chronic—not acute—conditions, dramatic cures are unlikely, and mysterious diagnostic challenges rare. "Treat 'em and turf 'em" or "Buff 'em and turf 'em" and on to the next "gomer" seems to be a growing popular hospital litany.

As we have seen in Chapter 7, community-based long-term care agencies can get involved in this foray when one of their clients is hospitalized or becomes an agency client while an in-patient. We say "can" because communication flow between professional groups is very problematic. Like social workers and discharge planners, case managers in the community may be the last of the last to know that a client has been admitted or discharged or both—all in the same day!

With community-based long-term care agencies, a patient/client status presents some interesting turf problems for social service professionals. Whose patient/client is he/she anyway? Who is responsible for coordinating a discharge and placement? Are hospital social workers responsible for postdischarge follow-ups on such patient/clients? Is anybody talking to each other in the first place? We have observed that often they are not.

Amid all this professional posturing stands (sits or lays) the elder patient.

The issue of professional autonomy not only includes the elder versus the professional but also profession versus profession. For example, a recent proposal to reform how home health agencies operate under Medicare calls for nurses, not physicians as is current practice, to certify and monitor eligibility as well as to develop the plans of care (Mundinger, 1983). In other words, make the nurses more professionally autonomous and relegate the physician to diagnostician and consultant. Incidentally, in this 200-page volume, the author, a registered nurse, discussing reforms in home care for the elderly, does not once mention the terms "social worker" or "social work".

It must be recognized that prejudices and jealousies exist between professions. For example, in a symposium on aging a physician advocated for multidisciplinary teams caring for the elderly. This team would be made up of specialists: namely, ". . . a doctor, public health nurse, or an R.N. experienced in long-term care, a sane (sic) social worker, and possibly an ombudsman, etc." (Elder Press, 1983). This physician's diction is revealing and one can probably recall stories from social workers who have had to deal with "insane" doctors.

Even within groups significant conflict exists. For example, within the community-based long-term care movement, conflict centers on the emphasis of "health" or "medical" services. One subgroup calls for establishing a continuum of care with "medical and social services." Another group wants the continuum to be made of "health and social services." The choice between "medical" and "health" is a conscious decision. It reflects ideological tenets about what role medicine will play in the continuum of care, emphasized in the first and de-emphasized in the second. Future debates about community-based long-term care will have to settle the philosophical positions implicit in this word choice. Given the fervor with which advocates hold their positions, the debate may need some modern day Nicene Council to resolve the word choice and philosophical differences.

All in all, it does not add up to one big happy professional family.

RESOURCES

Societal resources like individual resources are multidimensional. These dimensions may be further subdivided into components of a particular dimension. Resources may be fiscal and/or informational. Their relative natures and perceived importance depends upon interest groups' points of view.

In the fiscal realm there are issues surrounding more or less dollars, and dollars versus services per se. The more or less dollars argument is probably as ancient as human society. It is probably traceable to some elder *Australopithecus* reaching out and grunting for a piece of recently killed game he or she was too weak to help capture. Whether or not our supposed elder ancestor was given meat by a caring member of the hunting party, other group members disapproved, or a dominant leader interceded, is unknown. We do know, however, that this same debate on how to allocate resources continues to this day.

One can almost reconstruct the elements of that early political debate.

"Okay, we'll give the old Gray Face some nuts and berries, but no meat, it's too hard to get and there's not enough for us all anyway."

"No! Gray Face must help pick and carry the nuts and berries in order to get a share."

"Wait, what about the time Gray Face cared for the young while we were hunting, and nursed my serious wolf bite until I healed?"

"Stop! Old Gray Face is my comrade and I am the strongest and hunt the most game so Graycie gets all she wants."

"Oh, all right, but if there is a drought next season, we're going to put this matter to a vote."

And so it goes.

A social welfare resources argument can be conceptualized as existing along parallel continua that may or may not intersect. That is, from zero dollars provided to an identified aggregate up to the "sky is the limit." On the services side there may be only coupons for food or no out-of-pocket health care costs up to the whole gamut of human services that a society could provide. In this latter case the society would become the equivalent of an affluent caring daughter that provided support in all the activities of daily living.

When distributing scarce resources—and "scarce" is a very relative concept here—values enter into the equation almost immediately. How is it to be done? By what criteria?

For the elderly, there is age-versus-need as a criterion. If age is the only criterion, there are no means tests or needs tests, only a biological status. Examples of age only as a criterion exist in Social Security and Medicare.

Contrast this to a program example like In-Home Supportive Services under the Social Services Block Grant of the Social Security Act where need must be demonstrated.

Analytically speaking, the needs approach is bureaucratic and not efficient. Social welfare legislation with complex and stringent needs tests may also be thought of as social services workers' employment acts. Institutions and empires have been built upon an ethic that recipients of social support must be truly needy.

However, on the positive side, a determination of need is presumably more equitable in that scarce dollars go to the most needy.

An age-only approach, on the other hand, is neat and administratively efficient. At age 65, 70, or 80, one receives "x," "y," and "z"—no mess, no fuss. Age is at the same time necessary and sufficient to affect support. Age as causal, however, has one significant drawback: everyone receives resources regardless of need, elder cosmetics heiress and ill-impoverished widow alike. An age criterion per se is inequitable and probably not very effective as a means of targeting resources.

When focusing upon issues surrounding the distribution of societal resources, a question must also be raised regarding resources for research into the processes and problems of aging. Do we not need operational information, and what should be spent for the purchase of scientific information?

What is aging? What is human aging? Is there normal human aging—even strictly biologically speaking? What about aging in a social context? All of these fundamental questions, although passionately debated, remain essentially unanswered to this day. For example, although analytic frameworks abound, and there are five or six behavioral science explanations of human aging, no comprehensive scientific theory exists (Kart and Manard, 1976).

If pressed for an explanation of aging phenomena ourselves, we would probably opt for a dual biological/social-psychological one. That is, biological aging is the end point of the human life cycle and successful aging is based upon adaptation to a problematic environment. At the same time, this problematic environment is itself socially constructed and reflexive. One may characterize our reasoning as the problematic adaptation to symbolic interactions in a phenomenological context.

As the reader can readily see, we too suffer from the same befuddlement as our theory-building colleagues. A comprehensive explanation of bio-psycho-social aging simply does not exist.

For those of us whose feet are planted on the hard ground of caring for the aged needy, recommending and writing social policy, and producing results in the long-term care wars, a lack of information is both frustrating and frightening. Expending scarce resources to care for a valuable and fragile group of elders—and doing it by the seat of your pants—as most of our contributors have done at one time or another—is a very humbling experience.

For example, community agency directors described in Chapters 3 and 6 have found themselves launched into the twentieth century, dealing with esoteric informational needs and processing issues. Sophisticated instrumentation and high technology hardware/software have become the new tools of the helping professions.

All this reminds us of the lifetimes of work that still remain to be done. Scientific information itself requires resources, and the allotment and distribution of resources is essentially a political process.

POLITICS

Policies result from political processes. Political processes, in turn, deal with exchanges of power. In the political arena the media of exchange are money, resources, and votes. In this era of "special interests" politics one could conclude that money as distributed through "special interests" outweighs vague pledges or promised votes. In our analysis we take this set of political circumstances as a given—at least for the time being.

The political arena in long-term care can be divided into two unequal parts: providers and consumers. Providers include such groups as the American Medical Association (AMA) and its respective state associations and the American Hospital Association (AHA) and its respective state associations. Major organized consumer groups include the Gray Panthers and the American Association of Retired Persons (AARP). When examining Congressional hearings it becomes clear that providers outnumber consumer witnesses. This is to be expected since providers have well-organized and well-financed lobbies. What follows is that the elderly undergo a metamorphosis into the pathological domain and become "clients" and "patients" whose problems are to be taken care of and resolved by providers.

The elderly, as a countervailing political force, seldom have a major say in outcomes that directly affect them. The most dramatic counter example of their relatively passive political posture was during President Reagan's initial attempt to "reform" Social Security benefits. Unfortunately, this example of almost unanimous agreement on an issue with concomitant follow-through is rare, and understandably so for two reasons. First, the politics of the elderly are as heterogeneous as they are themselves. For example, for some the Gray Panthers are too liberal and militant; for others the AARP is too conservative. Most of the "old-old" elderly, 75 years and over, have probably never even heard of these two politically active groups.

The second reason deals with electoral participation. Although on the whole elderly participation is greater than the rest of the electorate, participation and activity decline with age (Hudson and Binstock, 1976). Consequently, the oldest and most frail of the elderly do not constitute an active and supportive constituency.

With the exception of Claude Pepper and a few other legislative champions, the elderly are at a distinct disadvantage when "wheeling and dealing" in the political arena.

THE "PROBLEM"

In summary, we believe that the problems of the aged are largely those that are socially constructed and reinforced by the current political process—and therefore open to a competing set of blueprints.

Given the existing social context of growing old in America, we further believe that social constructions that create an increasing loss of individual personal autonomy are the most serious problems faced by elder citizens. Whether created by failing health, diminishing income, decreasing social networks and social support, or myths about growing old that form values and repressive institutions, an ever shrinking social world ending finally in death is a fate experienced by too many elders who lack options and alternatives.

We believe that solutions to problems associated with biological human aging ought to take the form of preserving, protecting, and fostering personal liberty.

ALTERNATIVES

Different groups have formulated various alternatives to the existing long-term care system during the last ten years. Specification of a particular alternative follows how its authors define "The Problem." For example, some Federal policymakers view "The Problem" as rising expenditures. Consequently, capping Title XIX, thus limiting expenditures under Medicaid, was a major feature of one Federal alternative (USDHEW, 1978). If "The Problem" becomes "fragmentation of services" and the "irrationality" of the present system, then specifications of the alternative are different. In this case, the alternative takes the form of a "unified" system. Its authors call it a "social health maintenance organization" with the unappealing acronym of "S/HMO" (Diamond and Berman, 1981).

Others, who view "The Problem" from more of the economist's eye for market efficiencies, see the alternative built around increasing cash in hands of elders (Metzer, Farrow, and Richman, 1981). They believe that additional income will allow elders to purchase needed additional services. It follows that a "supply" of service providers will arise once this new "market" becomes established.

Another approach is to export "The Problem"—whatever it is. This is sometimes done under symbolic names such as "New Federalism" or "local control." A recent example is what happened to social services funded through Title XX of the Social Security Act. In this case, Title XX funds, which had been targeted toward certain categories of people and toward certain service priorities, became a block grant to the states. Virtually all program accountability, from the Federal point of view, was eliminated. All conflict surrounding the establishment of service priorities and the definition of program beneficiaries was exported out of Washington. Significant disparities already exist between the states in terms of services to the elderly (Estes et al., 1983). This "exportation" process is more like an abdication of Federal responsibility toward the elderly.

We could provide additional illustrations but we think the point has been made: fragmentary problem definitions will produce fragmentary alternatives. To be sure, these fragmented alternatives acknowledge problematic areas that are not their central problem focus. For example, the alternative of capping Medicaid expenditures also called for expanding home health services. However, its principal purpose was obvious: limit expenditures.

A mathematician, viewing all the problem definitions, might conceptualize the whole problem as made up of a set of simultaneous equations. That is, the specification of each aspect of the problem (e.g., housing, income, medical and social services, and transportation) must be made. Then, each individual equation, representing one problem, must be simultaneously solved along with the others. Such global solutions have been attempted.

For example, a perennial favorite is to combine Titles XVIII, XIX, and XX of the Social Security Act into one comprehensive payment and service structure. On face value, bringing together Medicare, Medicaid, and social services makes for an attractive proposition. But then what about income strategies through Title XVI's Supplemental Security Income (SSI) and the states' State Supplemental Payment (SSP)? And what about housing through Sections 8 and 202 of the Housing Act administered through the Department of Housing and Urban Development? And, last but not least, what about the effects of all this on the family which has traditionally been the principal caregiver to the elderly?

No doubt all the "and what abouts . . .?" lead those who develop alternatives to apply Ockham's razor to problem definitions and let the nicks fall where they may!

As the mathematician erases the set of simultaneous equations from the chalkboard, the political scientist reminds him or her that the American political policymaking process is incremental. Due to the complexities involved, global solutions are the exception, not the rule (Wildavsky, 1974).

From this general discussion, we can define five basic alternatives. All except one, the "National Social and Health Insurance Program," have been described in the long-term care literature (Callahan and Wallack, 1981). Since this alternative, as we define it, is new, we provide a detailed description as an addendum to this chapter.

After describing these five alternatives we evaluate them according to a set of criteria. We draw these criteria from our discussion about the constitutive elements of the problem in long-term care. They include such notions as personal autonomy, professional autonomy, and equity. We also assess the probability of the implementation of each alternative. Our "grading" of these alternatives is summarized in Table 10.1.

Status Quo (SQ)

The first alternative is "STATUS QUO." This alternative means that the major policies and way of doing business will remain in place. It also implies that minor changes may take place but that they will be incremental. Existing payment and delivery methods would remain the same.

Table 10.1 Ranking of Alternatives

Criteria	Alternatives				
	SQ	Community	S/HMO	NSHIP	INCOME
Autonomy:					
Personal	Low	Mid.[a]	Mid.	Mid.	High
Professional	Low	Mid.	High	High	High
Resources:					
Cash	Low	Low	Low	Low	High
Services	Low	Mid.	Mid.	High	High
Political Appeal:					
Consumers	Mid.	Mid.	Mid.	Mid.	High
Providers	High	Mid.	Low	Low	Low
Equity	Low	Mid.	Mid.	High	High
Efficiency	Low	High	High	Mid.	High
Probability of Implementation	High	Mid.	Low	Low	Low
Public Cost	High	Mid.	Mid.	High	Low

[a]Mid. = Middle.

Community-Based Long-Term Care Agencies (COMMUNITY)

The "COMMUNITY" alternative means a major expansion of the type of agencies that are described in the preceding chapters. These agencies would have more control over resources than would be allowed under the SQ. However, control of medical services would still be vested with physicians, typically not on agencies' payrolls. These agencies would be a significant adjunct to the SQ.

Current Federal legislation allows for the expansion of Medicaid financed community-based long-term care agencies. Under section 2176 of the Omnibus Reconciliation Act of 1981, states may apply for Medicaid waivers to establish local agencies. As of July 1983, 33 states had 43 waiver programs approved. Of these programs, 14 are directed toward the aged and disabled and an additional 13 programs combine the aged with other subgroups such as the mentally retarded (La Jolla, 1983).

Social Health Maintenance Organization (S/HMO)

The "S/HMO" alternative would significantly affect existing payment and delivery methods. Based on a uniform per capita payment and a prospective reimbursement schedule, these S/HMOs, as envisioned in our scenario, would develop on an ad hoc basis. In other words, their creation would depend on local conditions and preferences. Eligible populations would be determined locally. As with the community-based long-term care agencies, the S/HMOs could be an adjunct to the SQ.

National Social and Health Insurance Program (NSHIP)

It may be time to consider that the United States establish a "National Health and Social Services Insurance Program" for the elderly. NSHIP would be organized on the basis of federally run S/HMOs and staffed by salaried personnel. It would be funded on a capitation basis and all individuals aged 65 and over would be eligible at no cost. To finance this alternative, Medicare and other categorical programs for the elderly would be discontinued and their funds transferred to NSHIP. If these programs did not provide sufficient funding, then additional funds would be financed through Federal income taxes, not through payroll deductions.

A significant difference between this alternative and the others is that it would be national policy. It would replace the existing SQ.

Income Maintenance (INCOME)

The "INCOME" alternative can be conceived as directly transferring cash either in the form of actual payments or in the form of vouchers for services. For simplicity's sake, we define this alternative as consisting of cash grants available for home and institutional care. Under this alternative, the elderly would receive a monthly check for a fixed amount. Any expenses incurred would be 100 percent tax deductible; otherwise, the grant would be treated as taxable income and taxed according to the individual's own tax rate. This particular feature would introduce the notion of horizontal and vertical equity to this proposal. If a particular elder needed more services than the grant could purchase, then an assessment of need would be carried out, by the Social Security Office, for instance, and additional sums could be authorized. A monthly grant of $350 per individual would cost approximately $92 billion a year. This amount is roughly equivalent to cashing out completely Medicare and Title III of the Older Americans Act as well as a pro rata share of Medicaid, Title XX social services, and the SSI/SSP's cash grants.

CRITERIA AND GRADING OF ALTERNATIVES

Personal Autonomy

By "Personal Autonomy" as a criterion we mean that the alternative in question supports personal freedom of the elderly. The mechanics and internal policies of an alternative would be focused toward supporting, fostering, and protecting self-government.

Regarding "Personal Autonomy," the INCOME alternative receives the highest mark. This is so since the elderly would have cash in hand to "shop around" for needed services. We do not believe that a possible objection to this ranking, based on the questionable competency of the elderly to "shop around," is valid. Almost all studies which have investigated sources of support of the elderly point out that friends and family are the major sources of help. There are very few noninstitutionalized elderly who are absolutely alone. Consequently, if an elder becomes enfeebled, then friends and family will be able to assist in the purchase of needed services. Legal guardianship is always there as a last resort.

We rank the other alternatives, except SQ, as a "Middle" in terms of fostering "Personal Autonomy." Our reasoning for not giving them a higher rank is that although these alternatives do provide more options to the elderly they are essentially bureaucratic. For example, most community-based long-term agencies are presently marginal to the existing medical system. As such, they have to set up parallel and duplicative needs assessment and paperwork. It is not uncommon for an elderly person, served by such an agency, to be seen by seven different professionals as he or she passes from the hospital back to home.

S/HMO and NSHIP also receive a "Middle" ranking. We do so not so much because of increased bureaucracy but because these alternatives are based on a capitated prospective payment system. Due to economic incentives the elder's personal autonomy may not always be foremost in the minds of providers. That is, in-home care may be less expensive than inpatient care, but doing nothing costs less.

We rank the SQ as "Low" because of its institutional biases and lack of widespread options.

Professional Autonomy

"Professional Autonomy" means an increased sharing in decision-making. It also means less outside activities centered on process and more concern about outcomes. This implies less concentration on documentation and paper work and more attention to results.

We rank three alternatives as "High": NSHIP, S/HMOs, and INCOME. We do so because these alternatives do not place the physician in the central controlling role as under SQ. Due to the continued primacy of the physician in SQ, we give it a "Low." Our three "High" alternatives would allow for more shared decisionmaking and require less documentation and external regulation. We believe that this would come about in the NSHIP and S/HMOs alternatives because of economic incentives. Other professionals, nurses and social workers, could have more of a say in treatment decisions—and they traditionally advocate more in-home services rather than costly inpatient services.

Since COMMUNITY is still largely marginal to the medical model, we rank it as "Middle." Only through the determined efforts of the professionals in community-based care, as evidenced throughout this volume, do they make an impact on the medical decisionmaking process.

The INCOME alternative would also promote shared decision-making. This would come about because the elder, with cash in hand, would be more attracted to a physician who offers a "full range of services." Physicians would soon realize that the "demand" would be more toward a multidisciplinary "product" than just a medical "product."

Resources: Cash

In this context "Resources" means what effect a particular alternative will have regarding more or less resources: cash and services.

The only alternative which has as its objective increased cash in the hands of the elderly is INCOME. The other alternatives do not include cash as a benefit.

Resource: Services

Only the NSHIP alternative receives a "High" ranking as far as increased services are concerned. We say this since a full range of services would be mandated across the country. This would not mean that NSHIP would be financed with a blank check. Being dependent on Federal income taxes would make it somewhat budget conscious. COMMUNITY, S/HMOs, and INCOME receive a "Middle" ranking because we believe the expansion of services would be more dependent on local "market" conditions and on a particular area's capacity to generate a supply of services. This would be particularly true in rural areas. Current limited or nonexistent alternative services give SQ a "Low" rank.

Political Appeal: Consumers

Political appeal is another two-part criterion. First we make a judgment as to the relative political attractiveness of an alternative from the point of view of the elderly themselves as consumers. Then, we make the same judgment from the point of view of providers.

We think that the INCOME alternative would have the greatest political appeal to elders themselves. Cash talks and increased disposable income in the hands of the elderly would represent a significant shift in the existing power structure.

We rank all other alternatives as "Middle" given the heterogeneity of political attitudes among the elderly. We believe that each proposal would have sufficient support from significant numbers of the elderly, but that no one alternative, other than INCOME, would have overwhelming support.

Political Appeal: Providers

We believe that providers, particularly physicians and hospitals, would favor the SQ, given the proposed alternatives. All other alternatives either entail a change in payment—from fee-for-service to capitation—or a diminution in their existing power. We give COMMUNITY a "Middle" ranking in recognition that providers other than physicians and hospitals, such as nurses and social workers, would support this proposal.

Equity

Our "Equity" criterion concerns how different groups of elderly are treated (e.g., are all elderly equal or do the "most needy" deserve special treatment). For our purposes, equity not only means that all elderly are treated the same but that the "treatment" facilitates access to needed medical and social services in an equal fashion. Equity here means a "fair distribution of opportunities" (Blum, 1974) for medical and social services among the elderly.

With this definition in mind, we rank both NSHIP and INCOME as "High"; COMMUNITY and S/HMOs as "Middle"; and SQ as "Low". Since coverage under NSHIP and INCOME is universal and beneficiaries are treated equally, we believe that these two alternatives are the most equitable. We give a "Middle" ranking to both COMMUNITY and S/HMOs, but for different reasons. The COMMUNITY alternative assumes that its clients are recruited on the basis of some targeting criteria (e.g., the most frail or the most at risk). Consequently, although that subset of elderly, for example the "at risk," may be treated equally, the rest of the elderly do not have access to the offered services. Our judgment is also tempered by the operational ability of community-based agencies to "target" intake accurately and to know when to terminate clients. The first situation would mean that because of imprecise operational targeting criteria, community-based programs may serve some elderly who, in fact, are not at risk. These "false positives" would be consuming resources which would be more beneficial for the "false negatives," the truly at risk, who were not accepted as clients.

The second situation may arise when a truly at risk client is admitted as a client but kept on the program after the risk had passed. As with the other type of targeting error, this client would be consuming resources which would be more beneficial if given to elders truly at risk but not yet clients.

We give SQ a "Low" because of the existing inequities of categorical programs such as Medicaid and their injurious effects on the near poor who do not "qualify" for services.

Efficiency

Efficiency is a troublesome notion in any context and no less so here. What we mean by efficiency is simply whether an alternative is effective when comparing what it may produce with what it may cost. Since the "effect" of "effective" is increased personal autonomy, an alternative is highly efficient when its associated costs compare favorably to increases in personal autonomy.

We give "High" ranking to INCOME and COMMUNITY, and "Low" to SQ. We view INCOME as highly efficient since it puts cash in the hands of the elderly. It lets them decide how best to promote their own personal autonomy. Similarly, we rank S/HMOs as "High" since the capitation approach will provide direct economic incentives to seek the lower cost of care. Obviously this logic would not hold true if the cost of nursing home care were to drop significantly below the cost of home care, or if S/HMOs got greedy and began to dramatically increase enrollment without increasing staff and services.

We rank NSHIP as "Middle" even though it also is based on a capitation payment system. We believe that its potential efficiency would be diluted by queuing problems. That is, the elderly may have to wait for services. Without a price mechanism to allocate services, the only way to ration services will be to impose waiting periods. Although this argument may be applicable to the S/HMOs alternative, we do not believe it holds true to the same degree.

SQ receives a "Low" ranking here because health care costs continue to skyrocket with no clear positive effects on the debilitating impacts of chronic illnesses—the major threat to personal autonomy.

Probability of Implementation

As with all the other criteria, our assigned values as to the "Probability of Implementation" of a particular alternative are subjective. Given our particular point of view, the reader will notice a high correlation between how we rank this probability and how we rank the "Political Appeal" to providers. It should be noted that even though a particular alternative may be given a "Low" probability of implementation, it should not be discarded. It simply means that strategies for its adoption should be based on a long-run game plan. Also, some of these alternatives are not mutually exclusive. For example, it may be possible to combine SQ with COMMUNITY.

Public Cost

How might the foregoing alternatives affect public costs? For NSHIP, initial costs would be high and level off or decrease over time. INCOME would probably start low and remain relatively low depending upon the cost of living and inflation. Interestingly, competition between new entrepreneurial providers of community care (e.g., "Mother's Helper, Inc.") could actually reduce costs of in-home supportive services. They could further reduce public costs by keeping the frail out of hospitals and nursing homes and remove the need to "spend down" to a welfare status for Medicaid in-home services! As we saw in Chapter 9, becoming "poor on purpose" is sometimes the only alternative.

In addition, INCOME would eliminate the administrative overhead of existing programs. In this sense, INCOME would be an auditor's unemployment act.

SQ costs would likely remain in the current relatively high range. Since the inception of Medicare, health care costs have consistently been at the top of the consumer price index. Even with the advent of Medicare's DRGs, we suspect costs will continue to be high. One only has to open the professional journals to get advice about "How to Optimize DRGs." In this context, optimization is synonymous with maximizing revenues with creative diagnoses.

We rank COMMUNITY and S/HMO as "Middle" since, if they were implemented nationwide, we think that savings would eventually be achieved. It would probably take several years before the savings of in-home and preventative care were of the magnitude to be more than the additional administrative costs. However, in the long run, these two alternatives would be less costly than SQ.

DISCUSSION

In Table 10.1, no one alternative is clearly a "winner." Even if one alternative had all but one "High" out of our ten criteria, the subjective importance that one places on the exception may be such as to outweigh all the other criteria.

If one were to assign a point value to the "grades" to quantitatively rank each alternative (e.g., "Low" = 1; "Middle" = 2; and "High" = 3) and assume that all the criteria are of equal weight, then INCOME scores the highest. Even if it did not, our personal preference would still be for INCOME since, in our judgment, it provides the most toward the personal autonomy of the elderly—our central value.

Realistically, we recognize that this alternative has a low probability of implementation since providers, of all professions, would strenuously oppose it. In addition, mainstream American values generally react negatively to just "giving away money." So in our judgment, INCOME is not now a politically feasible alternative.

On the other side of the political coin, we think that the problems of equity and efficiency associated with SQ are such that its political support will eventually be eroded. In the face of this erosion an alternative will be chosen to replace the current way of doing business.

We believe that the chosen alternative will be COMMUNITY. A significant but still incremental change to SQ, COMMUNITY has the advantage of possessing the necessary characteristic of a politically feasible solution that the others do not: something for all parties. As we saw in the preceding chapters, elders definitely are much better off with community alternatives as are their families. The $100 billion "pot" we mentioned in the beginning of this chapter would be more equitably distributed among all providers. COMMUNITY would not seriously jeopardize the present hegemony of physicians. Legislators could point to these programs which they authorized as concrete examples of "doing something." Even sceptical fiscal curmudgeons can be given the hope of expected savings through the more extensive use of community-based care.

If all this sounds cynical, we should point out that the implementation on a wide scale of this alternative will require legislative support. Without a working majority and support from many quarters, legislators will not pick up on major new issues. Sometimes political realities engender cynicism.

With COMMUNITY, all institutional interest groups are represented and prosper by undertaking kinship tasks, as in the oldest and most fundamental institution of them all—the family. Our hybrid symbiotic relationship of kinstitution appears to be a concept and solution uniquely appropriate to the needs of our times.

COMMUNITY, as kinstitution, represents incremental compromise and is characteristic of the Western nation-state. A redeeming virtue of kinstitution (speaking to advocates of more dramatic social change) is the emphasis on society as responsible kin, society as communal and familial—even maternal. Kinstitutions hold a promise of further liberating women from the largely unrecognized and uncompensated labor of caring for the frail elderly.

All in all, because COMMUNITY does hold out something for everyone and because American society will no longer tolerate the injustices and inequities of the existing arrangement, we feel that community-based long-term care will soon be the norm rather than the exception.

ANTICIPATED AND UNANTICIPATED CONSEQUENCES IF COMMUNITY ALTERNATIVE ADOPTED

Peering into a crystal ball to predict the future is risky business at best. Our intention here is to speculate about a probable future, given that the incremental independent variable of case-managed long-term care emerges as dominant. This is not to say that other alternatives are not more desirable or will not coexist, or even become predominant, in some distant future. Rather, our ponderings reflect upon what appears to be a likely compromise in the ongoing long-term care wars, and what a supremacy of case-managed long-term care might change in everyday life. Whatever images we conjure up are in part due to changes brought about by significant demographic shifts.

Economic Effects

In an economic realm we see the development of spinoff suppliers of goods and services for homecare of the frail and disabled. For example, grab bars and raised toilet seats in hardware stores, compartmental and nonskid dishes in department stores (other than in the infant and children's section), and special clothing in dress shops (other than only through mail order catalogues) will become more prevalent. Like the authors, the reader, too, may have observed that underwear for incontinent adults and adult size "diapers" are now available in neighborhood supermarkets and regularly advertised on television.

If "case managers" become a significant employment group, we suspect that whole armies of social workers will evolve into case managers right out of M.S.W. graduate programs (schools of behavioral and social science will prosper also). We wonder if the title of social worker will become archaic and experience the same fate as stewardess (now flight attendant) as more and more men enter a burgeoning job market traditionally populated by women?

We are confident that if community-based long-term care prospers as a way of life, fewer and fewer young-old frail and inappropriately placed elders will be warehoused in nursing homes. This trend may have a major impact on housing. Pressures for low or moderate cost housing are strong even today and we only see the situation deteriorating.

One current and popular solution to housing shortages are underground, that is illegal, in-law apartments. We have observed such arrangements everywhere and they provide shelter for a surprising number of the elderly. One need only take a stroll down any R-1 rated street (Residential, single family occupancy) in San Francisco and count the separate side entrances, mail slots, door bells, automobiles, dog droppings, and parked shopping carts to obtain a hint of the magnitude of illegal "in-laws."

Another economic consequence of community-based long-term care that we predict involves a divergence in the flow of dollars from one part of the private sector to another. It stands to reason that if nursing homes lose their privileged status as the only major alternative for long-term care, those same care dollars will flow into different parts of the private sector as well as stay in the pockets of families that would have paid an average of two thousand dollars a month to keep a loved one in a skilled nursing facility! An example of this branching dollar flow again comes from our observation in San Francisco. A 94-year-old woman, Katie Hennessey, lives alone in an in-law apartment and although nearly blind, deaf, and frail, manages to live independently with the assistance of her brother, sister-in-law, and landlords. During the past months she has suffered one heart attack and two serious falls, resulting in deep wounds on her scalp and right elbow. Any one of these accidents would have put her into the hospital and probably nursing home were it not for the intervention of her extended family.

Katie's sister-in-law shops for groceries every Thursday evening and the landlord checks in every afternoon at five. The landlord's wife changes Katie's bandages daily and washes bedsheets after an "accident."

Katie neither saw a physician nor entered the hospital—she refused—following her injuries and was last seen happily scrubbing the bottom of a cooking pan after burning some canned tomatoes.

Dollars that would have been spent on Katie for doctors and hospitals were saved, thereby also saving Medicare dollars, while the landlord purchased a smoke alarm, shower nozzle hose, fire extinguisher, toaster oven, and new door mats. Katie's sister-in-law purchased a space heater, a small "electric broom" vacuum cleaner, and button-front dressing gowns. The landlord's sister-in-law purchased an exquisite crucifix as a gift on a trip to Italy and with that the community-based long-term care dollars flowed into the international monetary system!

Familial Effects

Community-based long-term care as a formal connection to the informal support system will in all likelihood have profound effects upon the social world of women. History is replete with examples of women as the less powerful caring for the powerless and marginal and looking after the interests of the destitute. Women have traditionally played important roles in the movements and conscience of American social welfare. With this in mind, we expect that gradual changes will occur (again) in the roles and statuses of women vis-a-vis the family and larger social structures.

We already know from our own research (Clark and Pelham, 1982) and current literature that women are primary and over-represented both as providers and as recipients of informal support.

Community-based long-term care could offer the opportunity for case managers to become more responsible and women caregivers less responsible for the day-to-day concerns of in-home care, if in-home supportive services flourish. We believe that family care providers will continue to be highly involved in the affairs of their loved ones, but the menial tasks will be undertaken by others. Concomitant with a lessening of daily drudgery will be the occasion to become an assistant case manager of sorts and become informed about the formal support system—no small task in itself!

We are of the opinion that if the support environment for a

frail elder becomes more nurturing and benign, so-called nuclear families could more easily extend themselves to maintain a stressful and needy member. Families could indeed be encouraged to become extended if tax incentives were provided for in-law apartments, for example.

Life forms, including homo sapiens, increase in numbers and longevity in a favorable environment, and we surmise that given a more advantageous social world, elders could adapt and remain vigorous and autonomous for a longer time. Meanwhile, families could themselves evolve, adapt, and prosper as their members age. Ideally, families would not suffer the stresses that force burnout, breakdowns, abuse, and eventually exclusion of overwhelming problem members, as presently happens.

Medical Effects

Our cited research on hospital discharge and placement decisions indicate that an implementation of case-managed long-term care could have significant, although gradual, effects on status quo medicine. The stories throughout this volume also attest to this effect.

We observed that hospital admissions, nature and length of stay, discharge, and placement are all affected by the intervening variable of a family member or friend. Our initial findings suggest that, given informal support, hospital admissions will be less frequent, discharge more timely, and placements to home. Such intervention often requires heroic efforts, as the natural flow moves inexorably toward the nursing home. In the absence of informal support, the case management team can provide this intervention, as we saw in Chapters 4 and 7.

In another dimension, we believe that the use and over use of drugs—particularly mind-altering drugs and depressants—will wane in desirability. This will occur for two practical reasons. First, if elders are living at home, the bias is toward clear-headed, independent living, not the quiet manageability desirable for a nursing home context. Second, if the elder is longer able to care for him or herself, the threat or reality of illness is pushed away by prevention. Also, as Katie Hennessey says, "You can never be turned into a zombie by an overdose of drugs if you stay out of hospitals and nursing homes!"

Finally, we foresee a less dominant, unilateral role for physicians in case-managed community-based long-term care. This is not so much because physicians will become active care team members, but because of an intervention into the patient/physician interface. Life-threatening situations that precipitate an acute episode will be negated (e.g., area rugs around glass coffee tables). When and if physician contact does occur, the patient will have an agent with a "stay at home" bias.

An enormous amount of work remains to be done.

COMMON SENSE AND POWER EXCHANGES

We believe that when all else fails, some common sense might come in handy. When talking "common sense," we want to keep in mind the central values we defined above. We also want to keep in mind the tension involved with these values. For example, the tension that exists between personal and professional autonomy. Our own values put personal autonomy ahead of professional autonomy. Consequently, our common sense suggestions are colored by that value.

This commonsensical approach leads us to ask elders what it is that they want. Listening to the stories and episodes in the preceding chapters leads us to believe that the elder, if asked, would say, "What do I want? I don't want to die in a nursing home." National statistics say that this is literally a rare event—hospitals are the most frequent place of death for the elderly—but the thoughts and feelings behind this statement are clear. Elders tell us that they want to remain autonomous and at home. Elders do not want to become victims of some medical-social complex which places organizational or professional goals or a "target income" above their own goals.

Another point is also clear from the stories in preceding chapters. Presently, it takes heroic efforts by both elders and professionals who support their autonomy to maintain their individuality and provide them with alternatives. Boundary crossing, as Chapter 5 graphically points out, is an exhausting activity. Common sense says that this should not be the case.

What is going on, as illustrated by the stories in the preceding chapters, is a power struggle. Exchanges of power are politics. Without being rooted in the political process and without the widespread political support of elders, any alternative is doomed to become a palliative to the majority and a boon to special interest groups.

ADDENDUM

A Description of a National Social and Health Insurance Program (NSHIP) Structure

Delivery of medical and social services would be done through a social and health maintenance organization. Each "Metropolitan Statistical Area," the U.S. Census' new term for the "Standard Metropolitan Statistical Area," would have at least three separate organizations to insure some freedom of choice and competitiveness. All social and medical services to the elderly would be provided through these entities unless an elder opted out for a private pay system.

Eligibility

All individuals entitled to a Medicare card would be eligible for this program. This means that the majority would be 65 years and older. It also means that some of the younger disabled population would be included. Given that these individuals also have sets of chronic conditions similar to the elderly, their inclusion seems appropriate.

In addition, although 97 percent of the elderly are covered by Medicare, three percent (approximately 700,000 individuals) are not. These individuals are typically persons with no Social Security income histories (e.g., Black domestic workers) or immigrants recently arrived in the United States who have not completed the mandatory waiting period for enrollment. To insure universal eligibility of the elderly, regulations affecting these two groups would be changed so that anyone aged 65 or over would be eligible.

Services

The whole continuum of medical and social services would be included. Individuals in the program would not need to undergo any other set of eligibility or "needs" determination.

Control and Internal Authorization

Administration of regional programs would be carried out by a typical management team consisting of department heads. Following current S/HMO models, social and other nonmedical services will have a more "status-equal" role in decisionmaking.

Fiscally competitive and maximally efficient programs will learn very quickly that acute days cost big dollars, so an emphasis will be placed upon in-home support—both for prevention and for earlier discharge. Over time, this obdurant reality will tip the balance of decisionmaking more and more toward social service community care.

Because of this fact, we anticipate that admission, length of stay, discharge and placement decisions, and social services levels will evolve from the idealized teamwork model currently described in the literature, to a real and operational teamwork decision necessitated by the bottom line. Specifically, allocation of resources within a S/HMO would become a team decision based upon efficient case management of client/patients. This means a more holistic rather than organ/disease approach.

Payment

The Federal government would be responsible for establishing a prospective capitated rate for service organizations. An initial estimate we make is $465 per month per eligible person or a total annual cost for the United States of approximately $139.5 billion. Keeping in mind the different funding sources that would be melded into this one funding mechanism (Medicare and proportionate shares of Medicaid, Title XX social services, and Title III social service) and the current expenditure levels of those funding sources, this represents an additional expenditure of approximately $60 billion. The increase is attributable to increased costs associated with case management and administration, approximately $200 per month per person.

Financing

Current publicly funded medical and social services are financed through a combination of payroll deductions (e.g., Medicare's Part A Hospital Insurance), general revenues from income taxes, both State and Federal (e.g., Medicaid and Title XX services), and private payments (e.g., Medicare's Supplemental Medical Insurance). We propose to continue this existing financing system. Additional revenues, needed due to expected increases in the eligible population, would be financed through general revenues and not through payroll deductions. We believe the latter method to be regressive and less equitable than the former. In the long run this will mean a "federalization" of long-term care because of the larger amounts collected through Federal income taxes. We believe this is preferred policy due to existing disparities between states in terms of levels of service that they provide to the elderly.

Personnel

NSHIP would be staffed by salaried personnel. Federal oversight would establish nationwide standards and minimum patient-to-staff ratios. Case managers would play a significant role.

Facilities

A National Social Health Insurance Program would serve as a vehicle to rejuvenate existing city and county hospitals and nursing homes. NSHIP would use these facilities as their primary sites of care.

Conjuring up a picture of a multipurpose social and health center with an energetic emphasis on outreach and community care—particularly a center that revitalizes county nursing homes—is warmly appealing.

REFERENCES

Blum, H. L. *Planning for health.* New York: Human Sciences Press, 1974.

Callahan, J. J., Jr., & Wallack, S. S. (Eds.) *Reforming the long-term system.* Lexington, Mass.: Lexington Books, 1981.

Clark, W. F., & Pelham, A. O. *Who is taking care of the poor old widows now?* Paper presented at the 1982 Annual Meeting of the Midwest Sociological Society Meetings, Des Moines, Iowa, 1982.

Diamond, L. M., & Berman, D. E. The Social/Health Maintenance Organization: A single entry, prepaid, long-term care delivery system. In James J. Callahan, Jr., & Stanley S. Wallack (Eds.) *Reforming the long-term care system.* Lexington, Mass.: Lexington Books, 1981.

Elder Press. Soquel, Calif.: The Elvirita Lewis Foundation, 1983.

Estes, C. L., et al. *Fiscal austerity and aging: Shifting government responsibility for the elderly.* Beverly Hills, Calif.: Sage Publishing Co., 1983.

Harris, R. *A sacred trust.* New York: New American Library, 1966.

Hudson, R. B., & Binstock, R. H. Political systems and aging. In Robert H. Binstock & Ethel Shanas (Eds.), *Handbook of aging and the social sciences.* New York: Van Nostrand Reinhold, 1976.

Kart, C. S., & Manard, B. B. *Aging in America: Readings in Social Gerontology.* Sherman Oaks, Calif.: Alfred Publishing Co., 1976.

La Jolla Management Corporation. *Analysis plan for Medicaid long-term care alternatives: Home and community-based care waivers and incentives for family care.* Prepared for the U.S. Department of Health and Human Services, HCFA Contract N. 500-83-0056, 1983.

Metzer, J., Farrow, F., & Richman, H. (Eds.) *Policy options in long-term care.* Chicago, Ill.: University of Chicago Press, 1981.

Mimnermos. In W. Barnstone (Ed.) *Greek lyric poetry.* New York: Schocken Books, 1972.

Mundinger, M. O. *Home care controversy.* Rockville, Md.: Aspen Systems Corporation, 1983.

Pelham, A. O., & Clark, W. F. *When do you go home: Hospital discharge and placement decisions for the elderly and implications for community-based long-term care.* Paper presented at the Thirty-Fifth Annual Meeting of the Gerontological Society of America, Boston, Mass., 1982.

U.S. Department of Health, Education, and Welfare. *Major initiative: Long-term care community services.* Memorandum for July 14 briefing. Washington, D.C., 1978.

Wildavsky, A. *The politics of the budgetary process.* Boston, Mass.: Little, Brown and Company, 1974.

Index